C0-FZI-791

HOSPITAL BUSINESS OFFICE

POLICIES AND PROCEDURES

Dudley Medlock, CPAM

D MED
CORPORATION

HFMA®
HEALTHCARE
FINANCIAL
MANAGEMENT
ASSOCIATION

TWO WESTBROOK CORPORATE CENTER
SUITE 700
WESTCHESTER, ILLINOIS 60154
TELEPHONE 708/531/9600

KENDALL/HUNT PUBLISHING COMPANY
2460 Kerper Boulevard P.O. Box 539 Dubuque, Iowa 52004-0539

HFMA gratefully acknowledges the gracious assistance of
Bobette Gustafson, Karen Hackett, and Pixie Hylton
in the content review of this book.

Copyright © 1990 by HFMA

All rights reserved. No part of this publication may be reproduced, stored in a retrieval system, or transmitted, in any form or by any means, electronic, mechanical, photocopying, recording, or otherwise, without the prior written permission of the copyright owner.

Printed in the United States of America
10 9 8 7 6 5 4 3 2 1

Library of Congress Cataloging-in-Publication Data

Medlock, Dudley.
Hospital business office policies and procedures/by Dudley Medlock.
p. cm.
ISBN 0-8403-5658-7 (Kendall/Hunt): $65.00 ($48.50 to members)
1. Hospitals—Business management. 2. Hospitals—Finance.
I. Title.
[DNLM: 1. Financial Management. 2. Hospital Administration—Economics. WX 157 M491h]
RA971.3.M44 1990
362.1'1'0681—dc20
DNLM/DLC
for Library of Congress 89-26928
CIP

HFMA BOOKS

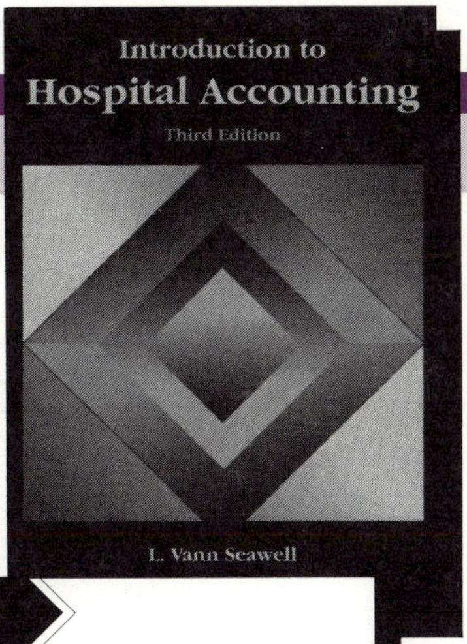

1992 Revised Edition!

Introduction to Hospital Accounting, 3d ed.

L. Vann Seawell, DBA, CPA

(See Page 8)

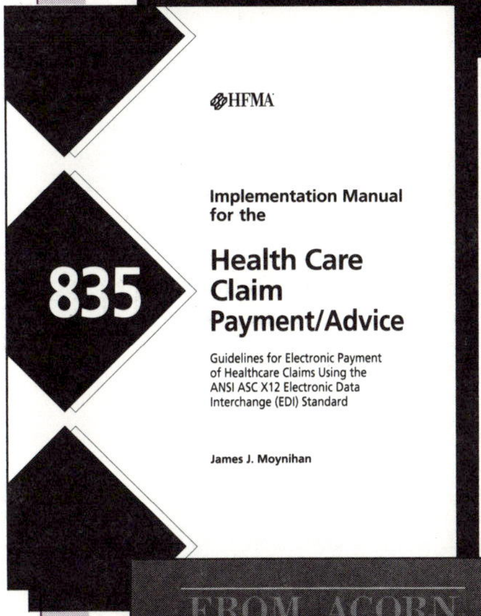

New This Year!

The Implementation Manual for the 835 Health Care Claim Payment/Advice

James J. Moynihan

(See Page 3)

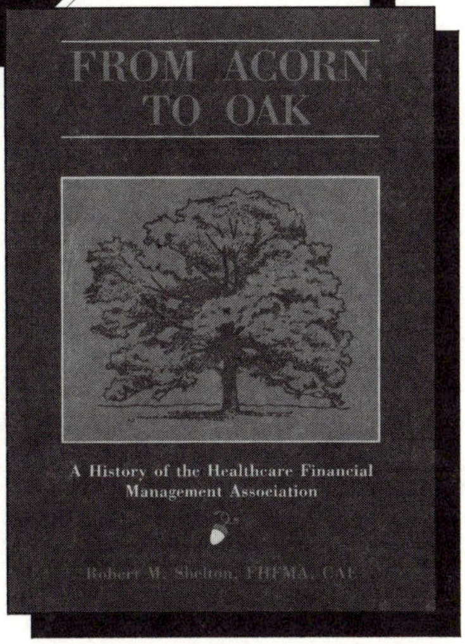

New This Year!

From Acorn to Oak: A History of the Healthcare Financial Management Association

Robert M. Shelton, FHFMA, CAE

(See Page 10)

Plus!
Three new guides for hospital trustees—Environmental, Antitrust, and Credentialing

(See Page 2)

Your best source for professional information to help you thrive in the 1990s

Healthcare Financial Management Association

SPRING 1992

HFMA® HEALTHCARE FINANCIAL MANAGEMENT ASSOCIATION
TWO WESTBROOK CORPORATE CENTER
SUITE 700
WESTCHESTER, ILLINOIS 60154
TELEPHONE 708/531/9600

Trustee Guide Series

HFMA BOOKS

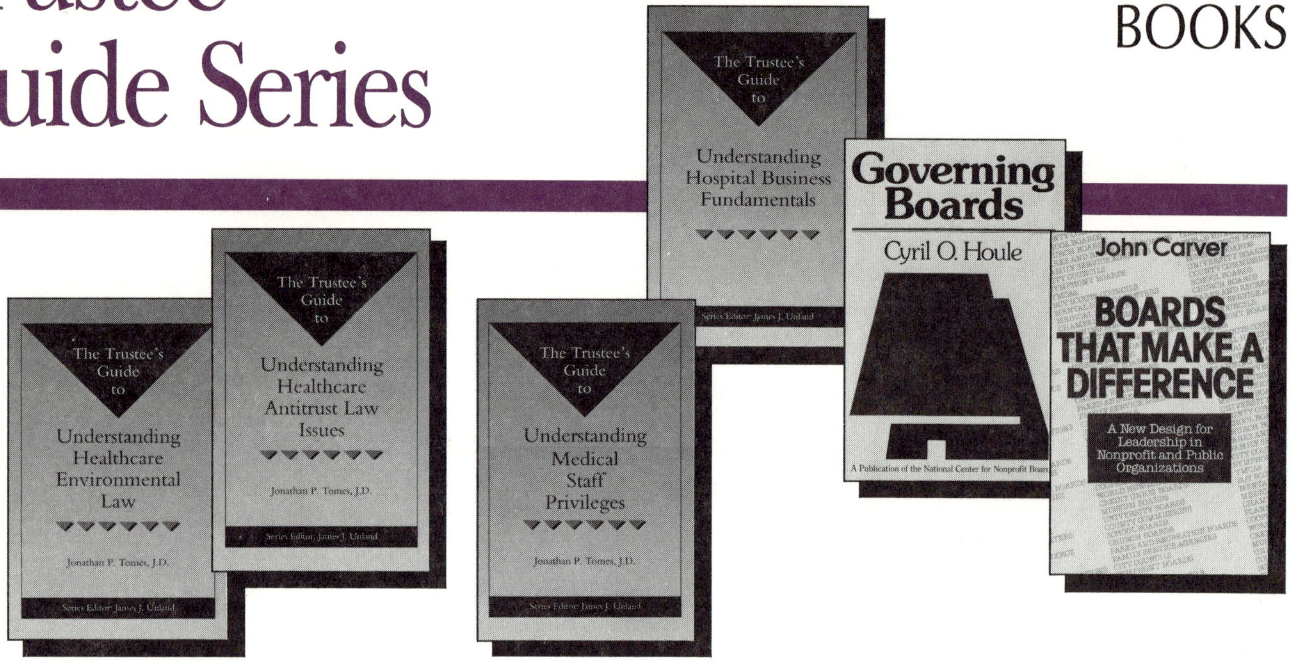

The Trustee's Guide to Understanding Healthcare Environmental Law

NEW

Jonathan P. Tomes, JD

This book will give hospital trustees an overview of the basics of healthcare environmental law. It will help trustees identify and examine the issues with respect to acquisitions and mergers, medical procedures, radiation, and medical waste.

ISBN # 0-930228-88-x

HFMA member price: $19.95
Nonmember price: $24.95
HFMA Order # 050161

The Trustee's Guide to Understanding Healthcare Antitrust Law Issues

NEW

Jonathan P. Tomes, JD

Hospital trustees can gain an overview of the basics of healthcare antitrust law issues using this book. Author Tomes clearly and logically outlines the many antitrust issues as they apply to healthcare organizations, especially hospitals.

ISBN # 0-930228-88-8

HFMA member price: $19.95
Nonmember price: $24.95
HFMA Order # 050162

The Trustee's Guide to Understanding Medical Staff Privileges

NEW

Jonathan P. Tomes, JD

This book describes the growing importance of proper hospital medical staff credentialing and examines the legal responsibilities of the administration, the medical staff, and the hospital trustees in credentialing issues.

ISBN # 0-930228-90-1

HFMA member price: $19.95
Nonmember price: $24.95
HFMA Order # 050163

The Trustee's Guide to Understanding Hospital Business Fundamentals

James J. Unland

Hospital trustees can use this book to learn the basics of hospital business management. Author Unland identifies and examines the issues trustees must face when participating in management decisions.

ISBN # 0-930228-81-2

HFMA member price: $19.95
Nonmember price: $24.95
HFMA Order # 050160

Governing Boards

Cyril O. Houle

JOSSEY-BASS PUBLISHERS

Drawing on the author's extensive experience in the field, this book skillfully demonstrates how to successfully handle the full range of challenges and problems facing board members.

ISBN #1-55542-157-1

HFMA member price: $18.95
Nonmember price: $21.95
HFMA Order # 050905

Boards That Make a Difference

John Carver

JOSSEY-BASS PUBLISHERS

This book presents a new model of board governance that challenges board members to build a strong, vibrant organization that achieves its goals. The author's approach enables boards to get down to the real business of governance.

ISBN # 1-55542-231-4

HFMA member price: $19.95
Nonmember price: $22.95
HFMA Order # 050906

HFMA® HEALTHCARE FINANCIAL MANAGEMENT ASSOCIATION
TWO WESTBROOK CORPORATE CENTER
SUITE 700
WESTCHESTER, ILLINOIS 60154
TELEPHONE 708/531/9600

ISBN Prefix 0-930228

Cutting-Edge Skills

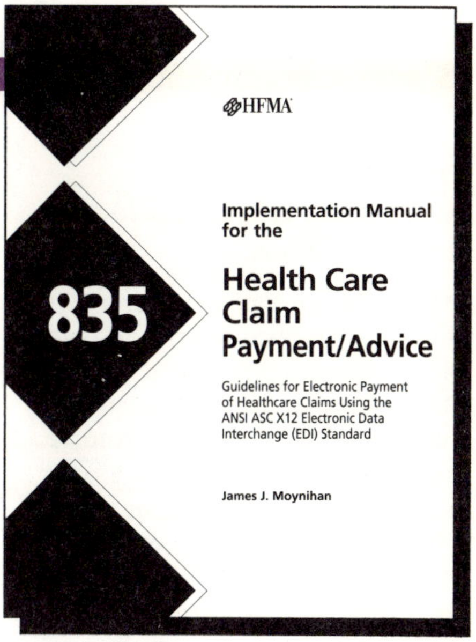

The Implementation Manual for the 835 Health Care Claim Payment/Advice NEW

James J. Moynihan

This is the official manual to the first nation-wide, all-payer electronic standard in health care, the Health Care Claim Payment/Advice (835). Use this standard to automate remittance processing. Committees of the American National Standards Institute (ANSI) developed the 835 standard. The author is the co-chair of the group that developed the standard. Part I, "Understanding the 835," will help those new to electronic data interchange (EDI) to understand the process. Part II, "Implementing the 835," includes all the technical information sophisticated EDI users need to mesh current patient accounting practices with the 835 format. Published in a three-ring binder for quick updating.

ISBN # 0-930228-91-x
HFMA member and
X12 Committee member price: $59.95
Nonmember price: $74.95
HFMA Order # 050230

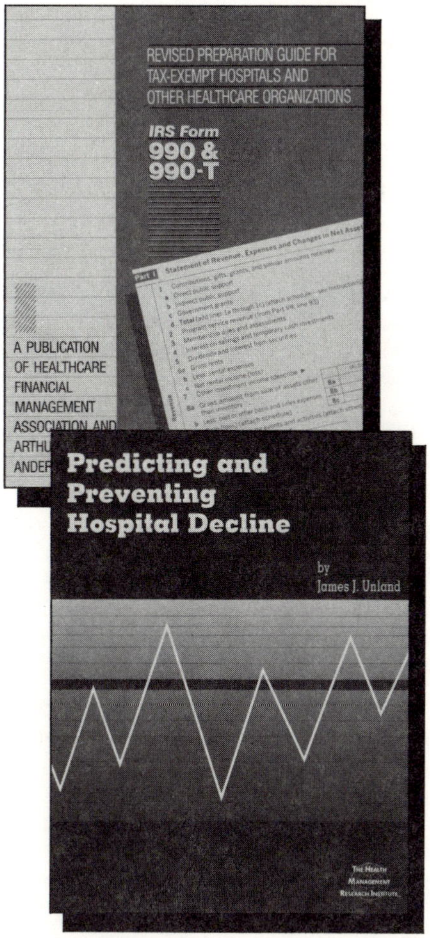

IRS 990 & 990T: Revised Preparation Guide for Tax-Exempt Hospitals and Other Healthcare Organizations

HFMA / Arthur Andersen & Co.

If your organization must file an annual Return of Organizations Exempt from Income Tax (IRS Form 990), this guide includes everything you need to expertly prepare your form for your institution.

ISBN # 0-930228-77-4
HFMA member price: $34.95
Nonmember price: $43.95
HFMA Order # 050150

Predicting and Preventing Hospital Decline

James J. Unland
HEALTH MANAGEMENT RESEARCH INSTITUTE

This book is designed to assist hospital administrators, board members, physicians, and department heads in identifying advance signs of trouble and correcting problems before they threaten a hospital's survival.

HFMA member price: $35.95
Nonmember price: $39.95
HFMA Order # 050912

To order, call our toll-free number, 1-800-252-HFMA, ext. 420.

HFMA® HEALTHCARE FINANCIAL MANAGEMENT ASSOCIATION
TWO WESTBROOK CORPORATE CENTER
SUITE 700
WESTCHESTER, ILLINOIS 60154
TELEPHONE 708/531/9600

Strategic Issues

HFMA BOOKS

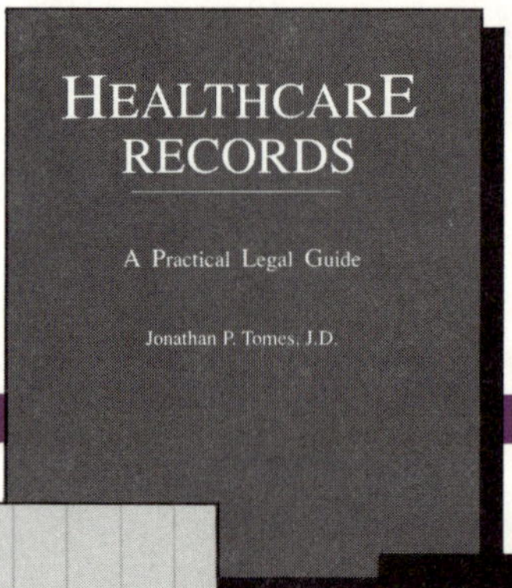

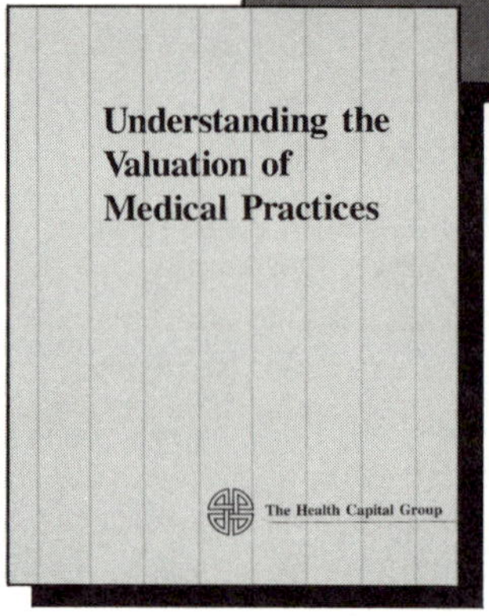

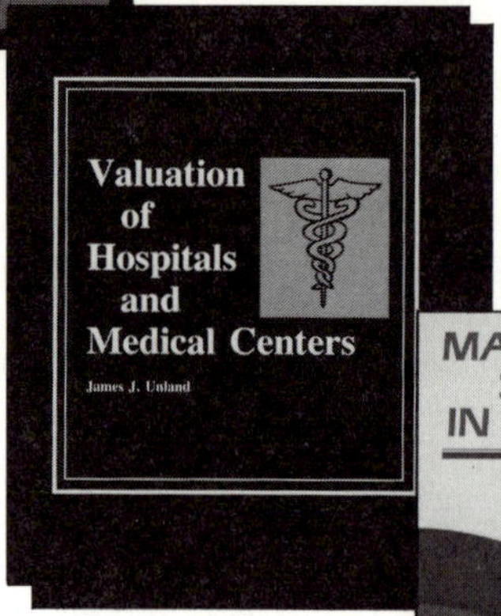

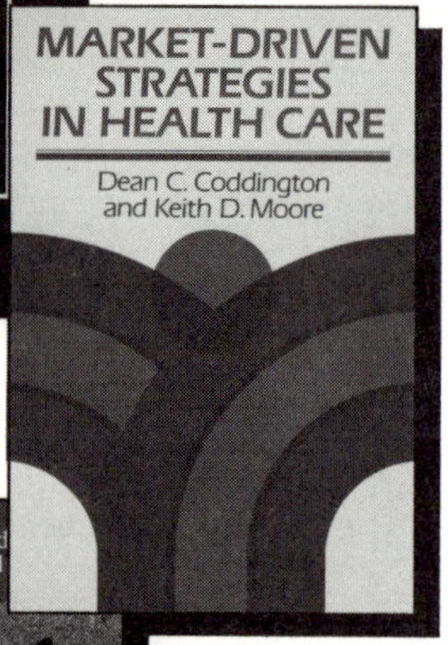

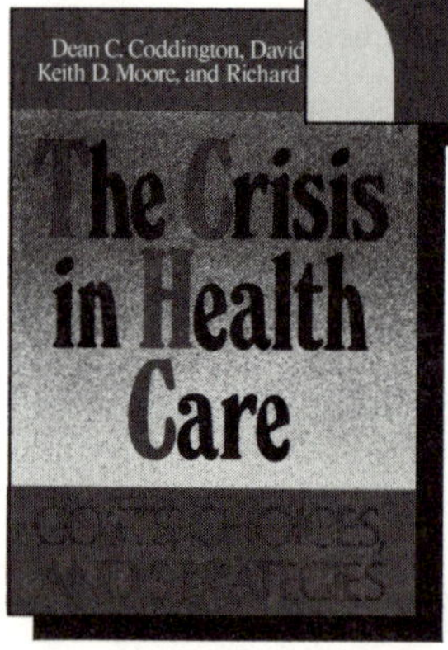

Healthcare Records: A Practical Legal Guide

Jonathan P. Tomes, JD

Written by a law professor for nonlawyers, this new book expands on the information in the former HFMA hospital records retention guide and will help you minimize your litigation losses, update your retention schedule, comply with the latest federal and state laws and regulations, protect your records, and streamline your records management system.

ISBN # 0-8403-5832-6
HFMA member $48.50
Nonmember $60.65
HFMA Order # 050060

Understanding the Valuation of Medical Practices

James J. Unland
THE HEALTH CAPITAL GROUP

This book helps healthcare financial managers understand how to valuate medical practices for both buyer and seller.

HFMA member $8.00
Nonmember $10.00
HFMA Order # 050901

To order, call our toll-free number, 1-800-252-HFMA, ext. 420.

Valuation of Hospitals and Medical Centers

James J. Unland
HEALTH MANAGEMENT RESEARCH INSTITUTE

This book will help healthcare financial managers, administrators, and trustees understand what they and their bankers must consider in valuating hospitals and medical centers.

HFMA member $34.95
Nonmember $43.95
HFMA Order # 050900

Market-Driven Strategies in Health Care

Dean C. Coddington & Keith D. Moore
JOSSEY-BASS PUBLISHERS

This book identifies the current and future needs of all three major healthcare markets (employers, physicians, and consumers) and outlines important competitive strategies, such as downsizing, networking, and others.

ISBN # 1-55542-045-1
HFMA member $29.95
Nonmember $37.50
HFMA Order # 050907

The Crisis in Health Care: Costs, Choices, and Strategies

Dean C. Coddington, David J. Keen, Keith D. Moore, and Richard L. Clarke
JOSSEY-BASS PUBLISHERS

Richard L. Clarke, FHFMA, President, HFMA, is one of the authors of this groundbreaking new book that offers strategies that payers, physicians, and providers can implement to survive the 1990s.

ISBN # 1-55542-273-x
HFMA member $25.95
Nonmember $30.95
HFMA Order # 050909

HFMA® HEALTHCARE FINANCIAL MANAGEMENT ASSOCIATION
TWO WESTBROOK CORPORATE CENTER
SUITE 700
WESTCHESTER, ILLINOIS 60154
TELEPHONE 708/531/9600

ISBN Prefix 0-930228

Patient Accounts Management

Hospital Business Office Policies and Procedures

Dudley Medlock

This book can help you increase your productivity, improve your cash flow, decrease your accounts receivable days, reduce your bad debt expense, and handle reduced staffing levels.

ISBN # 0-8403-5658-7
HFMA member $48.50
Nonmember $60.65
HFMA Order # 050050

Organizing a Healthcare Financial Services Division, 3d ed.

Russell A. Caruana, FHFMA

This significant revision incorporates major changes and updated material and continues the presentation of multiple organizational structures, titles, and job descriptions for various healthcare organizations.

ISBN # 0-930228-69-3
HFMA member $39.95
Nonmember $49.95
HFMA Order # 050110

Cashflow, Credit & Collection

Basil P. Mavrovitis
PROBUS PUBLISHING

A hands-on manual for general business applications complete with checklists, action plans, and practical case studies, this book demonstrates how an organization's credit function can be a profit center.

ISBN # 1-55738-078-3
HFMA member price: $19.95
Nonmember price: $24.95
HFMA Order # 050913

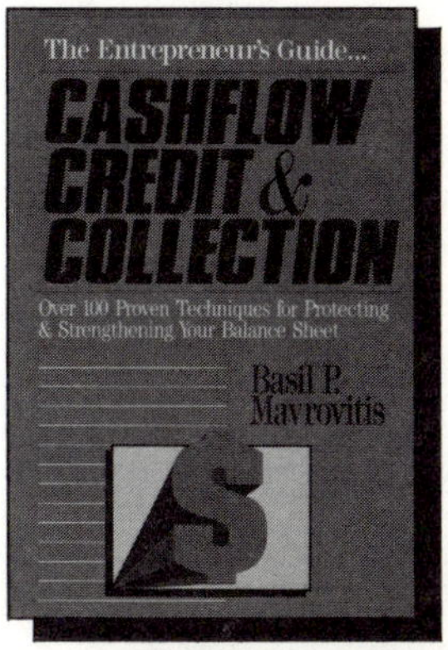

CP "Teach," 1992 Edition

Patrice T. Morin
MEDBOOKS

Buy a copy of this book for every member of your staff. They'll use it to improve their CPT coding accuracy and maximize reimbursement for the institution. And buy one for those doctors who have trouble filling out their portion of necessary forms.

ISBN # 0-923369-12-0
HFMA Member price: $31.95
Nonmember price: $39.95
HFMA Order # 050919

Supervision in Health Care Organizations

Richard I. Lyles, PhD, and Carl Joiner, PhD
JOHN WILEY & SONS

This basic text presents the fundamentals of supervision that nurses and allied health professionals need in positions of higher organizational responsibility.

ISBN # 0-471-80459-2
HFMA member $19.95
Nonmember $24.95
HFMA Order #050903

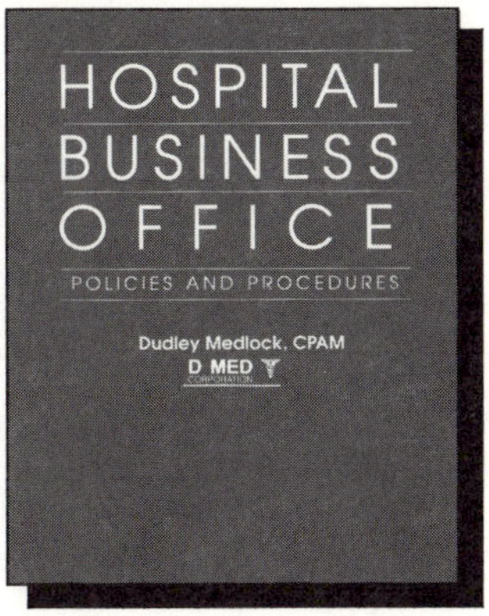

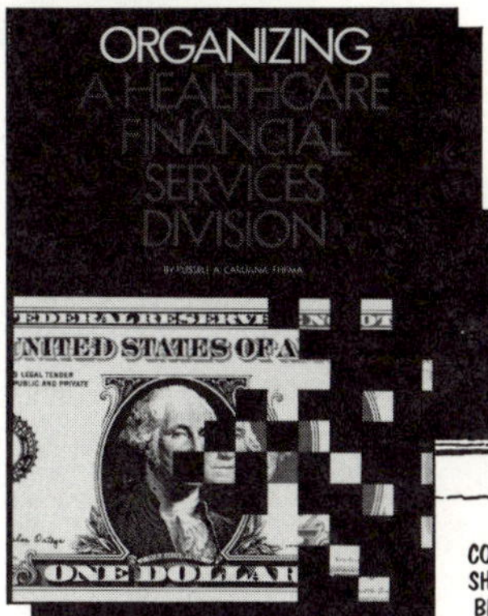

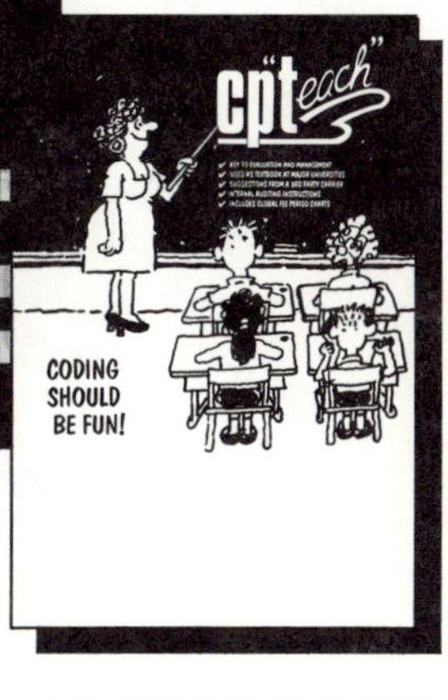

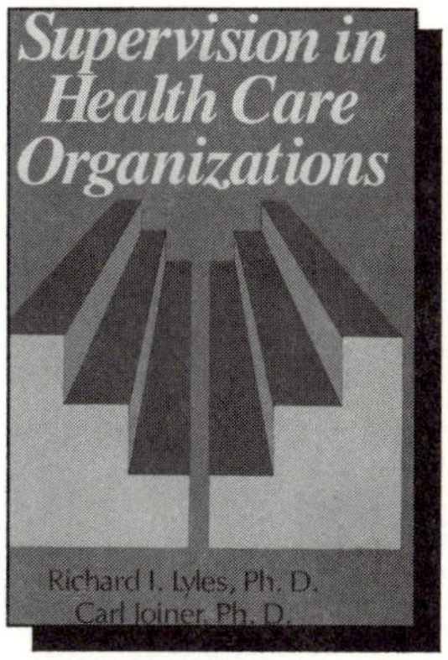

HFMA® HEALTHCARE FINANCIAL MANAGEMENT ASSOCIATION
TWO WESTBROOK CORPORATE CENTER
SUITE 700
WESTCHESTER, ILLINOIS 60154
TELEPHONE 708/531/9600

Professional Skills

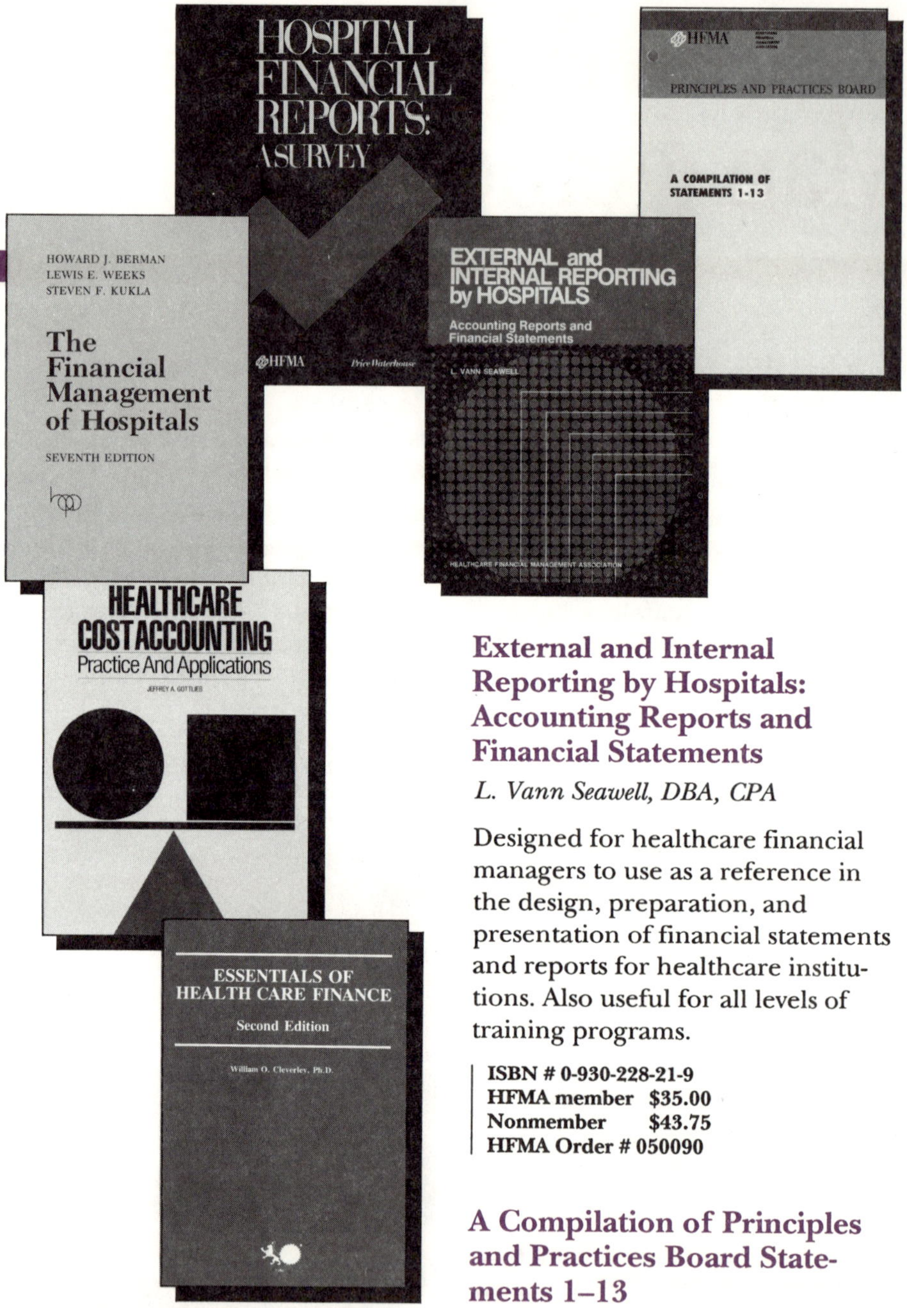

The Financial Management of Hospitals, 7th ed.

Howard J. Berman, Lewis E. Weeks, and Steven F. Kukla

HEALTH ADMINISTRATION PRESS

This revised and updated edition reflects the changing healthcare financial environment and makes it a more complete reference and text.

ISBN # 0-910701-53-7
HFMA member $55.00
Nonmember $68.75
HFMA Order # 050910

Healthcare Cost Accounting: Practice and Applications

Jeffrey A. Gottlieb

Written to make cost accounting less confusing and less mysterious by discussing the process and application, this book also provides details to help a financial manager immediately initiate cost accounting planning.

ISBN # 0-930228-67-7
HFMA member $29.95
Nonmember $37.50
HFMA Order # 050140

Hospital Financial Reports: A Survey

HFMA / Price Waterhouse

This book illustrates accounting trends, current developments, and areas unique to the hospital industry.

ISBN # 0-930228-52-9
HFMA member $29.95
Nonmember $37.95
HFMA Order # 050120

Essentials of Health Care Finance, 2d ed.

William O. Cleverley, PhD

ASPEN PUBLICATIONS

This revision emphasizes finance for healthcare firms in general, using illustrations from different healthcare sectors to develop major points.

ISBN # 0-87189-374-6
HFMA member $39.95
Nonmember $49.95
HFMA Order # 050902

External and Internal Reporting by Hospitals: Accounting Reports and Financial Statements

L. Vann Seawell, DBA, CPA

Designed for healthcare financial managers to use as a reference in the design, preparation, and presentation of financial statements and reports for healthcare institutions. Also useful for all levels of training programs.

ISBN # 0-930-228-21-9
HFMA member $35.00
Nonmember $43.75
HFMA Order # 050090

A Compilation of Principles and Practices Board Statements 1–13

HFMA Principles & Practices Board

The P& P Board believes that following consistent financial accounting and reporting practices makes for a clear understanding among the users of financial reports. Thus, the P&P Board has prepared the statements included in this report as guides.

ISBN # 0-930228-056-1
HFMA member $12.50
Nonmember $15.00
HFMA Order # 110009

HFMA® HEALTHCARE FINANCIAL MANAGEMENT ASSOCIATION
TWO WESTBROOK CORPORATE CENTER
SUITE 700
WESTCHESTER, ILLINOIS 60154
TELEPHONE 708/531/9600

ISBN Prefix 0-930228

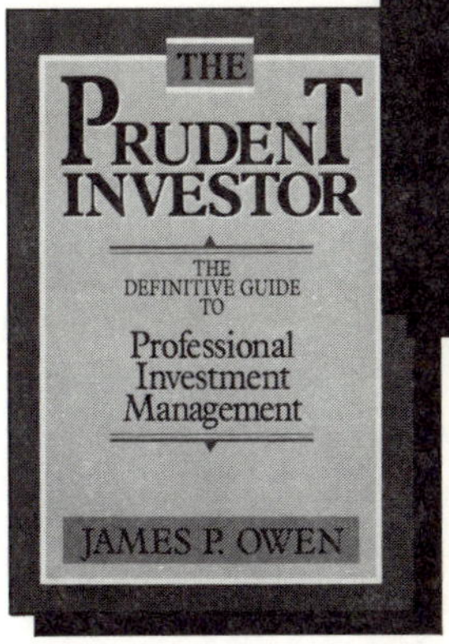

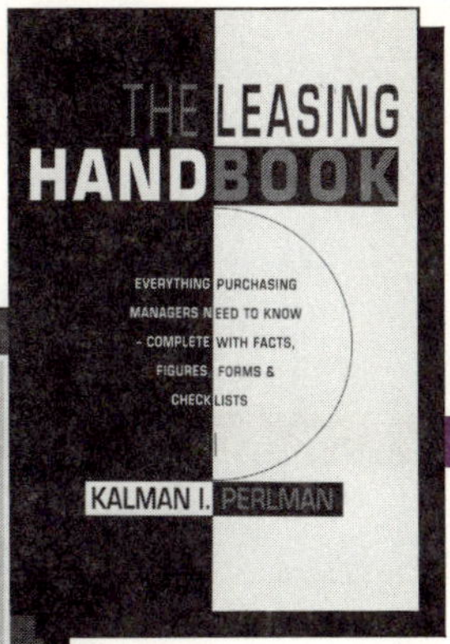

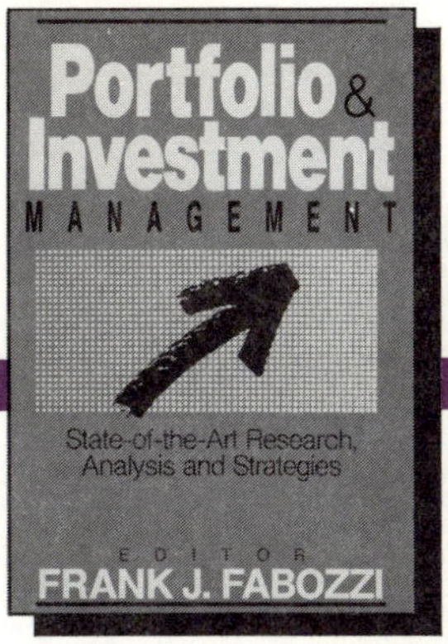

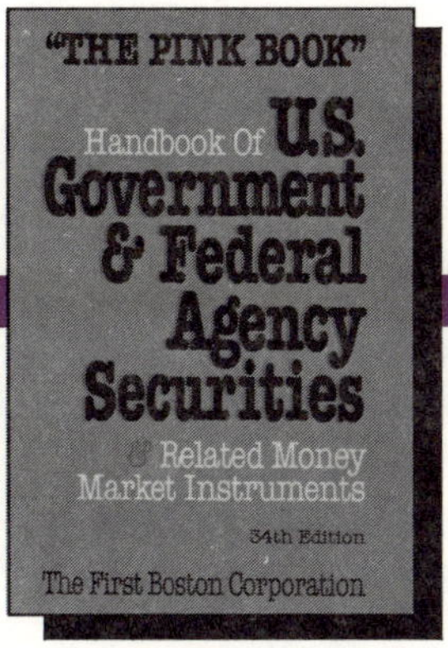

The Prudent Investor: The Definitive Guide to Professional Investment Management

James P. Owen
PROBUS PUBLISHING

A practical guide for the CFO who must now also manage the outside money managers. This book provides a master plan to improve the performance of the portfolio you manage: deliberately, incrementally, and consistently.

ISBN # 1-55738-106-2
HFMA member price: $22.00
Nonmember price: $27.50
HFMA Order # 050915

The Leasing Handbook: Everything Purchasing Managers Need to Know—Complete with Facts, Figures, Forms & Checklists

Kalman I. Perlman
PROBUS PUBLISHING

This book is the definitive guide to leasing for purchasing managers and others involved in acquiring capital assets.

ISBN # 1-55738-242-5
HFMA member price: $32.00
Nonmember price: $40.00
HFMA Order # 050914

Portfolio & Investment Management: State-of-the-Art Research, Analysis and Strategies

Frank J. Fabozzi, Editor
PROBUS PUBLISHING

Savvy investment managers who understand and apply the principles of portfolio management will be able to meet their risk/return objectives by employing a number of tools and techniques presented in this book. The editor gathered strategies, research, and analysis from contributing authors to help portfolio managers enhance the values of fund and portfolio assets.

ISBN # 1-55738-027-9
HFMA member price: $55.95
Nonmember price: $69.95
HFMA Order # 050917

The Handbook of U.S. Government and Federal Agency Securities: And Related Money Market Instruments, 34th ed.

First Boston Corporation
PROBUS PUBLISHING

Contains comprehensive and detailed factual information on the activities, instruments, and institutions of the U.S. Government securities market. The text also covers the futures and options markets for government securities, among many other things.

ISBN # 1-55738-168-2
HFMA member price: $23.95
Nonmember price: $29.95
HFMA Order # 050916

Discount and Return Policy for HFMA Books

Discounts

Libraries, bookstores, and college bookstores receive a 20% discount off the nonmember price. We accept stop orders. Individuals and other groups not mentioned here receive a 20% discount (off the member price for members and off the nonmember price for nonmembers) on orders of more than 25 copies of the same title.

Refunds and Returns

HFMA will accept returns only when HFMA has authorized the returns in writing before shipment of the books back to HFMA. HFMA will accept only returns accompanied by the following paperwork:

1. Copy of the signed return authorization from HFMA.
2. Copy of the invoice or packing slip from HFMA.

HFMA will not make refunds on damaged return items. HFMA accepts only returns that conform to this policy. If you have questions regarding discounts or returns, please call the HFMA Order Department at 1-800-252-HFMA, ext. 420.

Thank you.

HFMA®
HEALTHCARE FINANCIAL MANAGEMENT ASSOCIATION
TWO WESTBROOK CORPORATE CENTER
SUITE 700
WESTCHESTER, ILLINOIS 60154
TELEPHONE 708/531/9600

Textbooks

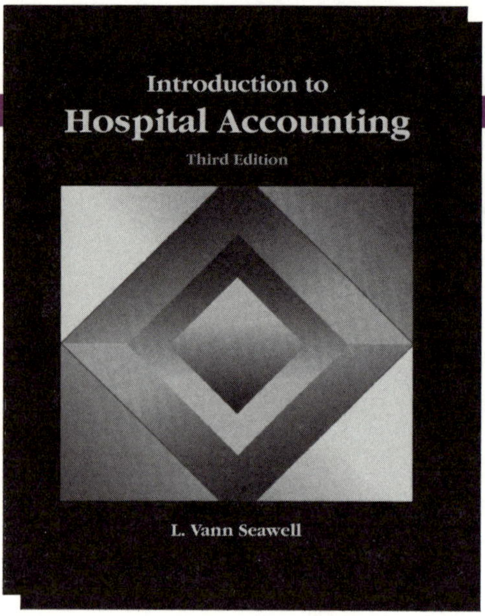

1992 Revised Edition **NEW**

Introduction to Hospital Accounting, 3d ed.

L. Vann Seawell, DBA, CPA
Professor of Accounting, Indiana University

Teachers, students, and working professionals will appreciate this updated edition of Seawell's perennial favorite. Each chapter of the book includes questions, exercises, and problems related to the chapter topic. It also includes a glossary of accounting and financial terms. Professor Seawell also has revised and improved the practice set and solutions manual to the text, both optional teaching aids.

ISBN # 0-8403-6310-9
HFMA member price: $49.95
Nonmember price: $59.95
HFMA Order # 050013

Table of Contents

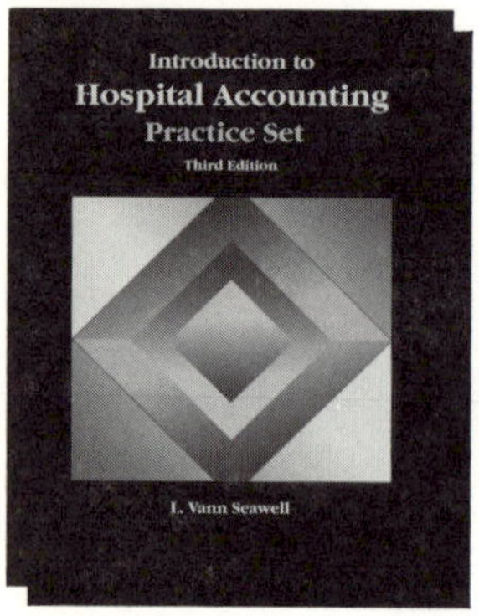

NEW

Practice Set

The new practice set is much more user friendly now. It's a workbook for ease of use and learning.

ISBN # 0-930228-94-4
HFMA member price: $54.95
Nonmember price: $65.95
HFMA Order # 050015

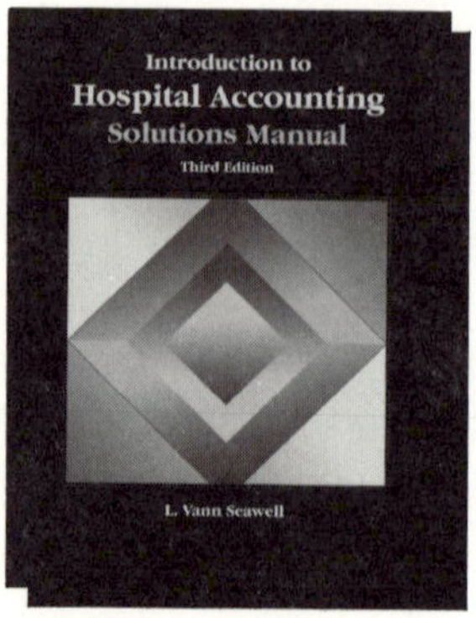

Solutions Manual **NEW**

The new solutions manual contains answers to the questions in the textbook and the solutions to the practice set.

ISBN # 0-930228-93-6
HFMA member price: $39.95
Nonmember price: $47.95
HFMA Order # 050014

HFMA® HEALTHCARE FINANCIAL MANAGEMENT ASSOCIATION
TWO WESTBROOK CORPORATE CENTER
SUITE 700
WESTCHESTER, ILLINOIS 60154
TELEPHONE 708/531/9600

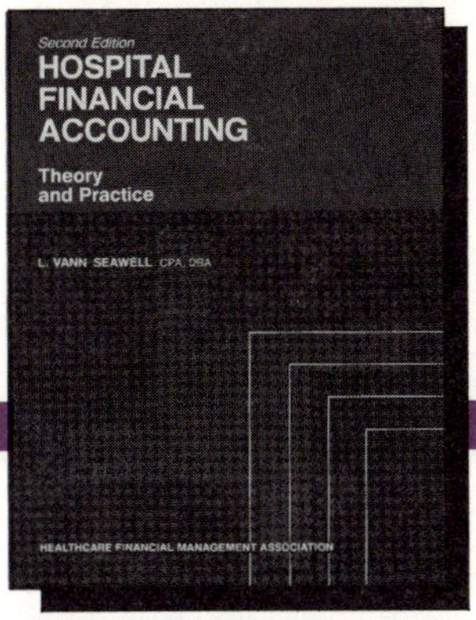

Hospital Financial Accounting: Theory and Practice, 2d ed.

L. Vann Seawell, DPA, CPA

This book is a useful general reference for anyone interested in the accounting and financial practices of hospitals. With emphasis on accounting theory and procedures, it also deals with related financial management. Instructor's manual is also available.

ISBN # 0-8403-4062-1
HFMA member price: $43.95
Nonmember price: $54.95
HFMA Order # 050020

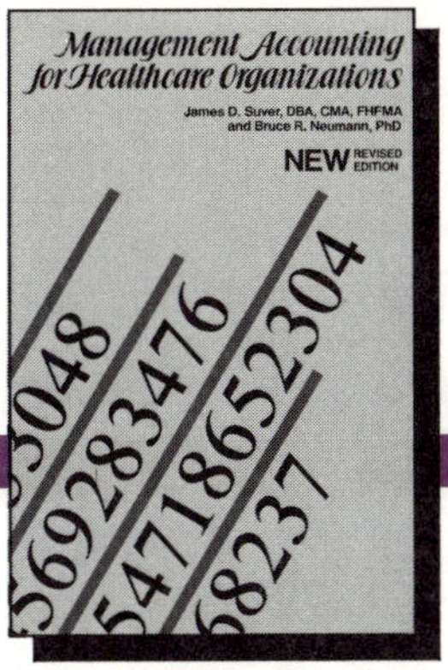

Management Accounting for Healthcare Organizations, 2d ed.

James D. Suver, FHFMA, DBA, CMA, and Bruce R. Neumann, PhD
HFMA/PLURIBUS PRESS

To order, call Pluribus Press, (312) 467-0424.

This text serves two distinct types of people: healthcare managers who need accounting information and accountants who need healthcare management information. Instructor's manual also is available.

ISBN # 0-931028-71-x
HFMA member price: $39.95
Nonmember price: $49.95

Coming soon!

Effective Patient Financial Services Management

Allen G. Herkimer

This revision of an Aspen book is expanded and updated to focus on the patient financial services manager of the 1990s. Author Herkimer also developed a workbook that accompanies the text for this improved edition of this guide to patient accounting. Expected to arrive in 1993.

New Revised Edition!

Management Accounting for Healthcare Organizations, 3d ed.

James D. Suver, FHFMA, DBA, CMA, Bruce R. Neumann, PhD, and Keith E. Boles, PhD
HFMA/PLURIBUS PRESS

The revised edition of this textbook will include an entire chapter on quality management issues for healthcare organizations to help the healthcare professional of the 1990s. Expected to arrive by fall of 1992.

To order, call our toll-free number, 1-800-252-HFMA, ext. 420, or use our order form on page 12.

HFMA® HEALTHCARE FINANCIAL MANAGEMENT ASSOCIATION
TWO WESTBROOK CORPORATE CENTER
SUITE 700
WESTCHESTER, ILLINOIS 60154
TELEPHONE 708/531/9600

Career Skills

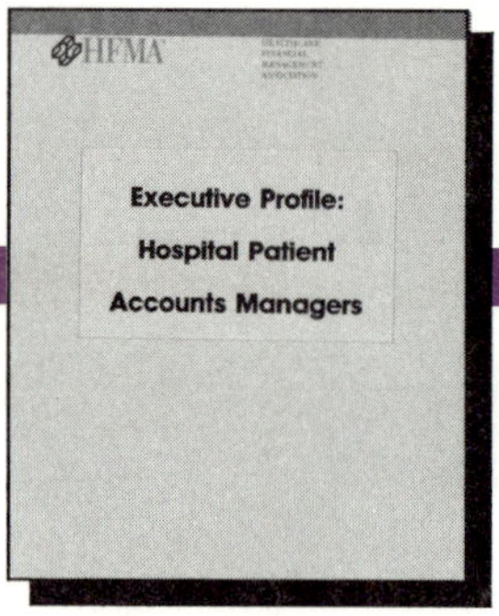

Executive Profile: Chief Financial Officers

HFMA / Witt Associates

Compare your situation to your peers' positions. *Healthcare Financial Management* journal regularly surveys the important chief financial officer position within HFMA's membership. This report, available in a loose-leaf binder so that you can add your own career information, offers an extended summary of the available data from the surveys.

ISBN # 0-930228-82-0
HFMA member price: $39.95
Nonmember price: $49.95
HFMA Order # 050201

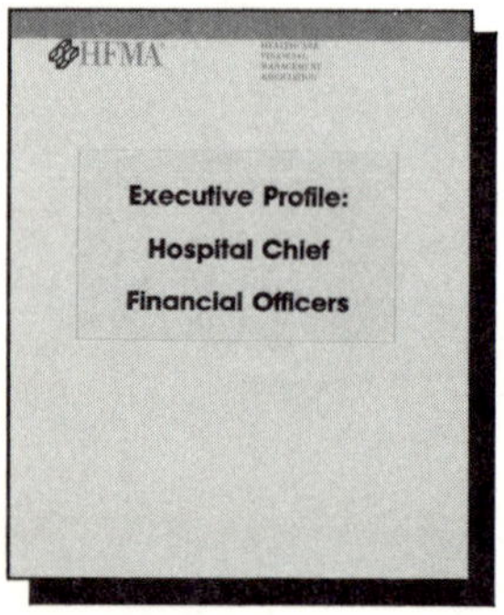

Executive Profile: Hospital Patient Accounts Managers

HFMA / Coopers & Lybrand / Accelerated Receivables Management Ltd.

Compare your situation to your peers' positions. *Healthcare Financial Management* journal regularly surveys the important hospital patient accounts manager position within HFMA's membership. This report, available in a loose-leaf binder so that you can add your own career information, offers an extended summary of the available data from the surveys.

ISBN # 0-930228-91-x
HFMA member price: $39.95
Nonmember price: $49.95
HFMA Order # 050202

New this year!

HFMA's independent study course. An at-home study guide. Improve your skills and test scores today!

Turning Health Care Leadership Around

Tom Atchison
JOSSEY-BASS PUBLISHERS

This book offers healthcare leaders practical insight into what motivates employees and how they form commitments. It will show how to lead an organization of self-managed, inspired employees dedicated to care.

ISBN # 1-55542-295-0
HFMA member price: $21.95
Nonmember price: $25.95
HFMA Order # 050904

From Acorn to Oak: A History of the Healthcare Financial Management Association

NEW

Robert M. Shelton, FHFMA, CAE

Author Shelton, a past executive of the Healthcare Financial Management Association (HFMA), traces HFMA's history from the philosophy of its original founders in 1946 up to the present day. Members will find the book an excellent insight into how changes in the healthcare industry affected the growth and direction of the Association. Community libraries will find the book an excellent resource for anyone wanting to know more about the healthcare industry and how the Association can help them to start a career in healthcare finance. (*Libraries—see our discount policy on page* 7.)

ISBN # 0-930228-84-7
Hardcover price: $39.95
Softcover price: $34.95
HFMA Order # 050243

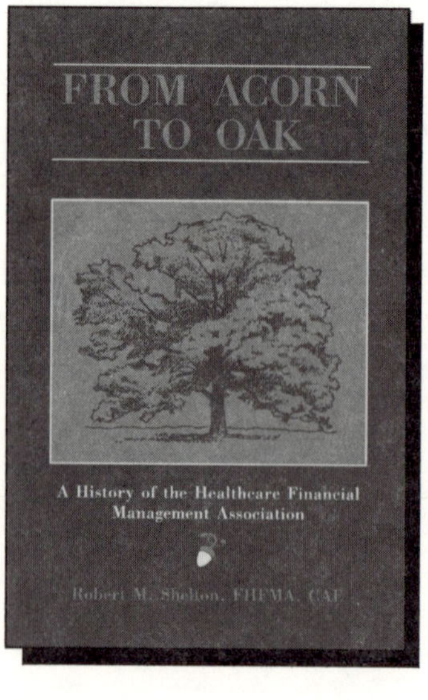

HFMA® HEALTHCARE FINANCIAL MANAGEMENT ASSOCIATION
TWO WESTBROOK CORPORATE CENTER
SUITE 700
WESTCHESTER, ILLINOIS 60154
TELEPHONE 708/531/9600

ISBN Prefix 0-930228

Certification

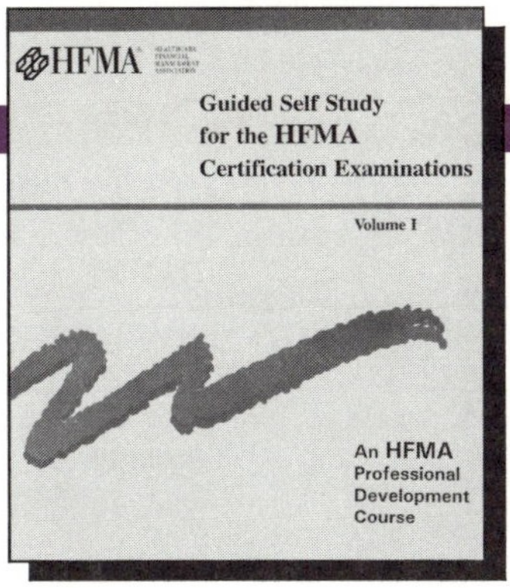

Certification Independent Study Course

NEW

Order this new course to prepare you for both HFMA's Fellowship (FHFMA) and Certified Manager of Patient Accounts (CMPA) exams, while you perfect the skills that you need to make it to the top of your profession. Gain points toward certification by completing the self-guided readings and by completing the accompanying practice tests.

HFMA member price: $195.00
(Discounts are not available on this book)
HFMA Order # 250020

The 1991/92 Certification Study Guides for the FHFMA and CMPA exams are required reading if you want to gain HFMA certification and advance in your career. Each guide contains sample questions, study bibliographies, and much more.

Fellowship Examination Study Guide

ISBN #0-8403-6005-3
HFMA member price: $45.00
HFMA Order # 250010

CMPA Examination Study Guide

ISBN #0-8403-6006-1
HFMA member price: $35.00
HFMA Order # 250015

Monographs

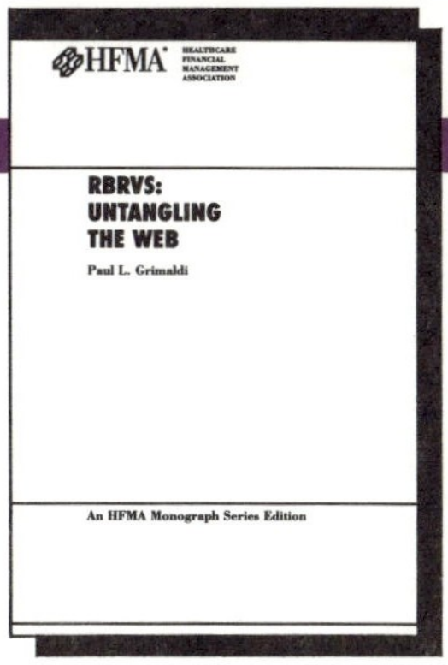

RBRVS: Untangling the Web

Paul L. Grimaldi

NEW

ISBN #0-930228-92-8
HFMA member price: $18.00
Nonmember price: $20.00
HFMA Order # 110011

The CFO's Expectations for Patient Financial Services

Vicki L. Romero and Judith B. Henry

NEW

ISBN #0-930228-87-2
HFMA member price: $15.00
Nonmember price: $18.00
HFMA Order # 110010

Fee Scale for Physician Services: Medicare's New Approach

Paul L. Grimaldi

ISBN #0-930228-76-6
HFMA member price: $8.00
Nonmember price: $10.00
HFMA Order # 110006

Capital Planning: A Leadership Tool for Chief Financial Officers

Kenneth Kaufman

ISBN #0-930228-66-9
HFMA member price: $8.00
Nonmember price: $10.00
HFMA Order # 110003

Data Services

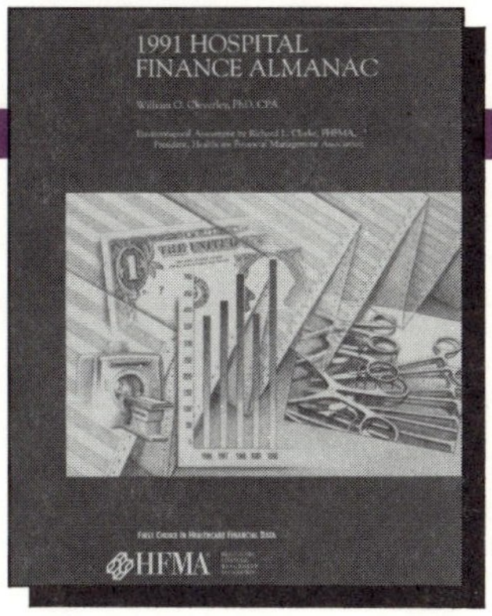

1991 Hospital Finance Almanac

NEW

William O. Cleverley, CPA, PhD

ISBN #0-930228-86-3
Retail price: $350.00
20% discount for libraries
HFMA Order # 222000

The *1991 Hospital Finance Almanac* is an annual publication that provides a comprehensive analysis of the financial and operating performance of the U.S. hospital industry. It includes data from 1986 to 1990 on the entire industry. The 1992 edition is expected in September.

Future Medicare Payment Alternatives

HFMA Task Force on Future Medicare Payment Alternatives

ISBN #0-930228-60-x
HFMA member price: $8.00
Nonmember price: $10.00
HFMA Order # 110002

Definition and Payment for Uncompensated Services and Special Problems of a Disproportionate Share

HFMA Task Force on Uncompensated Services

ISBN #0-930228-54-5
HFMA member price: $8.00
Nonmember price: $10.00
HFMA Order # 110008

HFMA® HEALTHCARE FINANCIAL MANAGEMENT ASSOCIATION
TWO WESTBROOK CORPORATE CENTER
SUITE 700
WESTCHESTER, ILLINOIS 60154
TELEPHONE 708/531/9600

ORDER FORM

When using this order form, please use the HFMA order number only.

Name

Title

Organization

Address*

City

State Zip + 4

Telephone

HFMA Member No.**

The above is my ❑ home ❑ business address.

Check, money order, purchase order number, or credit card information must accompany **all** orders. Telephone orders require purchase order number or credit card number. Shipping charges will be added for purchase order and credit card accounts. Prices and availability are subject to change without notice. Money-back guarantee. Please allow 2–4 weeks for your order to arrive.

* We ship UPS, so please use a street address.

** To get the member discount, please include your HFMA member number.

HFMA's ISBN Prefix: 0-930228

Quantity	Order #	Title	Price
		Total	$

❑ Total payment enclosed in the amount of $ ____________

❑ Purchase order # ____________

Credit card orders: ❑ VISA ❑ MasterCard ❑ American Express

Account no. ____________ Exp.date ____________

Authorized signature ____________

PHONE
1-800-252-HFMA
ext.420

FAX
708-531-0032

MAIL
HFMA Order Dept.
Two Westbrook Corporate Center
Suite 700
Westchester, IL 60154

Be sure to refer to HFMA's Discount and Return Policy on page 7 of this catalog

HFMA®
HEALTHCARE FINANCIAL MANAGEMENT ASSOCIATION
TWO WESTBROOK CORPORATE CENTER
SUITE 700
WESTCHESTER, ILLINOIS 60154

BULK RATE
U.S. POSTAGE
PAID
PERMIT NO. 2862
CHICAGO, IL

PLEASE ROUTE TO:

___ Chief Executive Officer
___ Manager/Patient Accounts
___ Chief Financial Officer
___ Manager/Receivables
___ Assistant Controller
___ Manager/Data Processing
___ Director/Patient Accounts
___ Supervisors

To the professionals
of patient accounts management

Contents

Detailed Contents

Preface

The purpose of this book is to provide a philosophy of management along with specific policies and procedures to help the professional patient account manager in today's complex world of patient accounts management. Intended to provide the tools necessary for an effective accounts receivable management program that the reader can adopt as is or modify with minimal effort and expense, the book has two parts. The first section outlines business office operations, providing a basis for understanding how an accounts receivable program works and how to process an account from beginning to end. The second part consists of specific policies, procedures, forms, accounts receivable management reports, productivity reports, and job descriptions. Intentionally, this book duplicates some information from one section to another and within the same section to provide the reader easy access to pertinent information relevant to various areas of patient accounts management.

This book emphasizes a fundamental approach to achieving management by exception rather than crisis management. Business Office Managers who implement this approach will note increased productivity, improved cash flow, decreased accounts receivable days, reduced bad debt expense, and reduced staffing levels. The book deals with the basic philosophy of controls and monitoring that is the very lifeblood of successful patient account management today.

For those who may take exception to the philosophies presented throughout this book, ask yourself this question: "Do I really know whether my current operation is efficient and effective, and how am I going to improve it?" If you can honestly answer the question, then you are probably already using some of the philosophies discussed in the book and can use the information discussed to excel in your profession. If you can't answer the question, you probably need to reconsider your current approach and begin applying the basic principles described throughout the book.

The approach and philosophies discussed aren't necessarily the one and only method for achieving excellence in the field of patient account management, but they do work. They are not fancy, but perhaps fanciness has contributed to the recent dramatic rise in accounts receivable. Some patient account managers seem to have been trying to use "whistles and bells" and forgotten about the basics.

Good luck in your endeavors to implement and maintain an efficient and effective business office and accounts receivable management.

Dudley Medlock

Dallas, Texas
April 1990

I

An Operations Overview

1

Pre-registration and Pre-admissions

Definitions

Pre-registration—the process and confirmation of patient demographic and financial information at least twenty-four hours in advance of arrival.

Pre-test—the diagnostic medical testing of patients in advance of registration to determine hospitalization and/or surgical suitability.

Suggestions for Implementing a Pre-admission Program

A pre-admission program can be started in a matter of days, and in some cases, a matter of hours with only a rearrangement of priorities and perhaps a few schedule changes.

Chances are that enough information is already available to allow pre-admission of 40%–50% of the next two weeks' admissions.

Recommendations for Implementation

Ask the Operating Room Supervisor for a copy of scheduled surgeries. Often a physician's office will call the surgical department of a hospital to put the patient on the surgical schedule, and will not notify anyone else. Establish a procedure whereby surgery will take such information, for scheduling purposes only, for the admitting office.

For the OB unit, ask the Nursing Supervisor for the pre-registration list, orientation tour list, and registration lists for Lamaze classes.

Visit primary OB physicians' offices weekly and obtain a copy of their registration sheets for new patients.

Give consideration to introducing the pre-admission program by sending a letter prior to the pre-admission representative's calling patients.

NOTE: Physicians should always be apprised of admission procedures and requirements.

Once these steps have been taken, there should be a less hectic atmosphere in the admitting office. A program that will enable pre-admission of other patients to the facility can be started.

> *When beginning a pre-admission program, concentrate on maximizing pre-admissions of scheduled surgery patients and OB patients first.*

Full Scale Implementation

To involve the maximum number of patients, the pre-admission program should be developed in three stages:

- Preparing the program.
- Selling and implementing the program.
- Monitoring the program.

Preparation

In preparation, a complete but simple outline of the intended operation of the program and its anticipated accomplishments should be created. If an informational pamphlet or pre-admission mailer is to be used, the preparation stage is the time to prepare these materials. The Patient Pamphlet, while not necessary in starting a pre-admission program, is a useful tool. This is simply an information booklet that may be given or sent to prospective patients. Take care to avoid overburdening the patient with information. The mailers can be made easy to understand by asking only necessary questions, and easy to mail by having the postage pre-paid. The mailer should emphasize that this procedure is for the patient's convenience and ask that the forms be returned to the hospital admitting office as soon as possible.

Selling

Selling the program is a vital step in assuring the program's success. A common misconception is that pre-admission is a complex and time consuming procedure. Emphasize that no new tasks will be added; the program requires only a change in the sequence of events.

The basic steps in selling the program are

- Presentation of the program to hospital administration to enlist their support.
- A medical staff meeting attended with the Administrator and Chief Financial Officer. The Administrator should take the lead in presenting the program and pointing out advantages to the physicians of prospective pre-admitted patients. Physicians will not be sold on the idea of a pre-admission program if only the potential benefits to the hospital are discussed; the benefits to physicians and patients should also be emphasized.

The following are some typical benefits a hospital can use to "sell" the program to physicians.

- Establishes personalized service for patients while enhancing continuity in the hospital admitting office procedures.
- Helps develop better public relations because of better understanding and planning by all parties concerned.
- Enables the business office to schedule arrival times and thereby maximize utilization of personnel and minimize delays for arriving patients, resulting in fewer complaints.
- Prevents long waiting periods for patients—those who have been pre-admitted will be taken before others.
- Prevents backlogs in admitting because of limited amount of time it takes to complete the admission process. Patient will sign necessary forms and proceed to the room. The total process should take no longer than five minutes as opposed to approximately eighteen to thirty minutes if not pre-admitted.
- Guarantees the patient a bed when the time comes to be admitted.
- Gives physicians a better opportunity to have the desired accommodations for their patients and the patients a better opportunity to receive the types of accommodations they desire.
- Gives preference to private room requests for pre-admitted patients.
- Verifies third-party coverage before admission. The patient, the hospital, and the physician's office will be aware of insurance benefits in advance, which will avoid any potential surprises to all parties concerned.
- Notifies physician's office of incidents of previous bad debts.
- Improves ability to screen patients financially. The hospital and the physician will have time to research sources of financial help when necessary.
- Improves ability to accurately estimate and collect deposits, which facilitates the hospital's issuing a courtesy discharge to the patient.
- Gives patients time to familiarize themselves with the hospital policies so that they will not have to face a mass of policies, rules, and regulations at admission.
- Gives patients time to become acquainted with the general layout of the hospital.
- Gives patients the opportunity to have the relaxed privacy of their own homes to fill out the information.
- Gives patients time to make any needed arrangements for their households.
- Provides additional direct telephone lines with recording devices installed in the admitting area to reduce the waiting time for physician office staff.
- Assists physician office personnel in setting up the desired follow-up system.
- Assists other areas in scheduling, such as dietary, lab, x-ray, and housekeeping.

These are just a few suggestions for selling the program. Do not, however, make promises you can't keep.

- Train admitting office personnel and emphasize the advantages of the program to the overall operation of the admitting and business offices. Many pre-admission programs have lacked effectiveness because personnel were not trained in telephone communications techniques, deposit computations, etc.
- Present the program to the Director of Nursing and O.R. Supervisor, stress its importance and request their full support.
- Recognize the most critical "Target Market" in selling this program. Physicians' nurses, secretaries,

and clinic managers can make or break the program. It is, therefore, essential that their support and enthusiasm be enlisted. Listed below are some ideas for gaining support.

- Hold monthly "get acquainted" breakfasts or luncheons with members of key physicians' staffs as well as hospital employees. Pre-arrange seating so that hospital employees sit next to physicians' employees and are able to communicate informally. During the luncheon, the Business Office Manager should always take time to point out the positive aspects of the pre-admission program and to thank everyone for their participation.
- Hold contests and present monthly awards to physicians' office personnel for the highest percentage of eligible patients who were pre-admitted. Such contests help to promote enthusiasm and show appreciation for their efforts.
- Offer to assist training physicians' personnel, and ensure that someone from the admitting office spends time helping with the pre-admission program.

Monitoring

A successful pre-admission program requires ongoing attention. The following suggestions are examples of helpful strategies that have been successful in the past.

- The Business Office Manager or a qualified designee visits the offices of key admitting physicians at least once every two weeks. These brief visits are designed primarily to promote and maintain the rapport between the business office and the physician's office. During these visits, any problems can be corrected quickly and the supply of pre-admission forms can be replenished.
- Keep accurate records of the number of pre-admissions filed by physicians and percentage of pre-admission mailers returned. Care is taken to identify "opportunities" for pre-admission rather than looking at total number of admissions requested by physician. For example, a physician admitting only OB patients has almost 100% opportunity for pre-admission, while an internal medicine physician normally has a lower percentage.
- Hold training meetings for business office employees at least monthly to reinforce procedures and discuss results.
- Hold contests among hospital personnel for the highest percentage of computed deposits collected or for improvement in quality assurance program scores.
- Continue breakfasts or luncheons for business office and physicians' office personnel. The guest list is varied, the pre-admission program promoted, and attendants thanked for their participation.

Some Common Objections to Pre-admission

- It's been tried before and it didn't help reduce receivables.
- The doctors using the hospital will not cooperate.
- There is no support from Administration.
- There is a census problem, so the hospital can't afford to push the program.
- There are not enough people in the admitting office to handle such a program.
- There is no time to develop a "patient pamphlet."

Responses to Objections

Objection # 1—Response

If properly administered, a pre-admission program will definitely improve receivables. When this objection is raised, it is usually because the program consists only of calling the patient and asking name, address, and type of coverage. A complete program includes the following:

- Adequate inservice training.
- Gathering all the necessary information and completing the admission form.
- Noting third-party coverage and verifying coverage by telephone.
- Calculating the deposit required based on admitting diagnosis and advising patients of deposit requirements prior to their arrival at the hospital.
- Explaining all financial requirements and other related information to the patient prior to entering the hospital.
- Screening patients to determine if there is a financial risk, and classifying patients by method of payment.
- Completing patient financial records.
- Reviewing completed pre-admissions by the Director of Admissions or the Business Office Manager.

Objection #2—Response

It is true that a number of physicians either do not wish to participate in a pre-admission program or simply do not have the time or personnel to do so. The following suggestions should help.

- Explain the program to the physician's office staff and try to ensure they are involved with it. As mentioned previously, the key to the success of such a program is the physician's staff. Develop a rapport with the physician's office personnel, and resolve minor problems before they become major obstacles. Once physicians are aware that their patients are spending less time in the admitting office, experiencing fewer cancellations, have better scheduling, have fewer complaints over financial requirements, etc., they will be much more supportive. Clearly, it is important to provide the physician with this information on a regular basis.

- Emphasize this key point: If procedures are well planned, the physician's staff will eventually spend less time communicating with the hospital admitting office.
- Inform patients when they enter the hospital that they should ask to be pre-admitted if they ever need to use the hospital again.

Objection #3—Response

Administration should play a major role in initiating the program, presenting the advantages to the medical staff and supporting the established written procedures on a day-to-day basis. It is ultimately the Administrator's responsibility to ensure effective implementation of the pre-admission program. The Business Office Manager should attempt to put together a complete program to sell to administration and keep reselling.

Objection #4—Response

Census should not be affected by a good pre-admission program. If it is, this usually means that a hospital has poor admission procedures and policies overall.

Objection #5—Response

A pre-admission program should not require additional staff since there are no additional duties, only a rearrangement of task completion times. In fact, some hospitals have been able to alleviate the rush of normal daytime hours by calling in the evenings and utilizing part-time employees to send mailers, set up pre-admission files, etc. The outpatient and E.R. registration clerks on the evening and late shifts can often be utilized for this function.

Objection #6—Response

It is not necessary to develop a complex patient pamphlet to start the program. Establishing policies, training personnel, and informing patients of required procedures during the patient interview will sufficiently initiate the program.

Mail and/or Prepare Pre-admit Form

Pre-admission mailer forms may be used if the reservation is made far enough in advance.

One method that can work successfully if the hospital has at least seven days' notice is to place pre-admission forms in the physicians' offices.

The pre-admission form can be given to the patient by the nurse or office staff when the reservation is made.

Design the pre-admission form with an information section that can be torn off by the office staff and sent to the hospital to notify the admitting office of the pending admission. The information section may then be filed in a tickler file with follow-up scheduled for three days from date of receipt, so that if the pre-admission mailer has not been received, admitting personnel can call the patient to complete the admission over the telephone.

Procedures

The admitting physician's office will call the hospital operating room staff or registration office to provide the following:

- Patient name, address, and telephone number where the patient can be reached, and social security number
- Patient age and gender
- Insurance information, including pre-certification or other special requirements, as applicable
- Physician name and telephone number
- Expected registration date
- Admitting diagnosis and expected procedures (i.e., specific invasive operative procedures-operating room, or non-invasive operative procedures-treatment room, etc.)
- Pre-test (laboratory, radiology, etc.) that will be performed as ordered by the physician

The information provided by the physician's office is keyed in to the pre-admission screen and a copy printed to begin the patient account file. In facilities that do not have on-line admission, the appropriate pre-registration form is manually completed.

The Utilization Review Coordinator is contacted for all Medicare beneficiaries requiring PRO approval of procedure prior to room assignment, and notified immediately of all Medicaid admits for completion of the proper authorization, when required.

Contact the patient immediately on receipt of the reservation.

All demographic and financial information is confirmed or added to the reservation form during contact with the patient.

Documentation is included in the patient account file for all contact with prospective patients to include no less than the following:

- Date
- Time
- Substance of contact
- Initials of registrar who performed the contact

Employment and insurance benefits are verified with the employer or insurance company once the pre-registration form is complete.

- Pre-certification, if required, must be obtained.
- Special requirements, as appropriate, must be identified.
- Insurance coverage must be clearly defined and documented for the type of service provided.
- Exceptions or limitations of insurance coverage must be documented on the verification form so the deposit requirement can be clearly defined for the patient upon arrival. This information is relayed to the patient through the second telephone call of the pre-admission process.

The registration deposit is calculated and documented prior to the second call to the patient.

The registration form is fully completed once all the demographic and financial information has been gathered and verified.

The pre-registered patient account file should contain the following information:

- Pre-registration form
- Patient contact documentation
- Insurance benefit verification
- Registration form completed, awaiting patient signatures upon arrival

The completed pre-registered patient account file is placed in a holding file under the expected registration date.

- The pre-registration holding file consists of a file drawer with dividers (1–31) representing the days of the month.
- The patient account file is placed behind the divider representing the day of the month for the expected registration date.

A pre-admission log is maintained. It indicates each patient's name, date expected, patient account number, and whether the insurance verification was performed. The Director of Admissions checks the log daily to ensure all pre-admits scheduled to be treated have had all necessary paperwork completed prior to the scheduled date of admission.

Review Pre-admission

Once the pre-admission is completed, the file is given to the Director of Admissions or the Business Office Manager for review and approval. This will ensure uniformity in the pre-admission process and prevent potential problems from developing on arrival of the patient.

Communication of Financial Requirements

Once the deposit requirements are determined, the patient is contacted again by telephone and advised of this requirement. Patients are asked to bring the deposit with them when they come for admission or, if time allows, to pay installments up to the time of admission. OB patients are advised that the deposit is required to be paid in one lump sum or in monthly payments, with the full amount to be paid by the end of the seventh month of pregnancy.

Prior to discussing financial arrangements, a "Credit Bureau Report" can be obtained. This report will provide additional insight into the patient's history of meeting financial responsibilities.

Financial Classification and Screening

At this point, it should be known what method of payment the patient intends to use. That is, the account can be properly classified as Medicare, Medicaid, Blue Cross, private pay, worker's compensation, commercial insurance, etc. For patients with no third party coverage (self-pay patients), pre-admission procedures offer the opportunity to determine whether the hospital is facing a potential loss. Subject to the policies established by the hospital, several possible alternatives will need to be explored prior to the patient's arrival for admission. These alternatives may include: referring the patient to social service agencies for assistance, consulting with the admitting physician and possibly referring the patient to another facility, or accepting payment arrangements for amounts to be paid after the hospital stay.

In every case, it is important to establish a complete understanding between patients and the hospital as to the patients' financial responsibility prior to their actual arrival at the hospital.

Determine Finances of Patient if No Third Party Coverage

The extent of the patient's ability to pay can be determined immediately by obtaining and confirming bank references and employment. If adequate resources are not available, the patient is encouraged to apply for Medicaid or available third party sources. Hospitals having social service departments should make this a part of their daily functions.

Determine and Collect Advance Deposits

If it is determined the patient must pay a substantial amount of the hospital charges, the amount due from the patient for the estimated stay is calculated and the responsible party is advised of this amount to be paid prior to admission. If the patient is a worker's compensation liability or other type case involving legal ramifications, the attorneys and the insurance companies involved are contacted immediately to determine how the account will be settled. Liens and other legal claims are initiated as quickly as possible if this course of action is necessary.

Admitting and Credit Coordinate to Resolve Problems

The admitting and the credit collection functions should work closely to investigate and verify the insurance coverage and financial status of a patient. This is especially true when there has been some indication that problems may be encountered in billing and collecting the amount due. If patients indicate during the telephone conversation that they cannot comply with any of your requests, the question should be resolved at this time. For example, if the patient cannot meet the deposit requirement, the admitting office should immediately notify the Business Office Manager and, with the patient, arrive at some mutually satisfactory arrangement. If one cannot be made, the physician should be called by the Business Office Manager, apprised of the situation, and asked if the admission can be delayed.

In some cases, administration may deem it appropriate to admit the patient due to the circumstances evident at the time. The Administrator, Chief Financial Officer, or other designated person authorizes such admissions, in writing, on the admission form.

Admission Forms

Initiate and prepare the following forms prior to the day of admission:

- Admitting Facesheet—the guarantor information should be complete and the guarantor signature obtained.
- Insurance Billing Information—would include Blue Cross, Medicare, commercial insurance, etc. The information completed would, of course, be only that patient data known at the time.
- Consent Form.
- Patient Charge Plate—if applicable, this would refer to the Addressograph or Elliott type card.
- Financial Agreement—outline of agreement on financial arrangements (e.g., $150 paid on admission and balance not covered by insurance paid at discharge).
- Memo Card or Follow-up Sheet—to be used by billing and credit department for follow-up and/or bad debt record.

Arrange the forms in an orderly manner for each patient with notations indicating what is to be accomplished when the patient is finally admitted.

Complete the preparation of admitting forms for all elective and generally all urgent patients prior to the time of admission. Only the admitting paperwork for emergency admissions will need to be done at the time of admission. If all possible pre-admission work is performed, more time and emphasis can be placed on special action for resolving problems and processing emergency admissions where investigations and confirmation of insurance coverages, etc., must be performed quickly.

From Pre-admission to Admission

At the time of pre-admission, certain procedures are initiated and followed through during the patient's stay until the time of discharge. Again at the discharge point, other actions commence immediately and are followed up closely in order that billings will be prompt, the collection follow-up effective, and the settlement of accounts receivable timely.

The pre-admitting/admitting personnel and their functions are vital to the overall successful operation of a hospital. They are generally the first hospital staff encountered by the patients; and quite often, the impression the patient gets at this point is the one that will be carried throughout. A bad impression puts additional strain on other hospital personnel, whose duties are difficult enough without any added burden caused by a disgruntled patient.

Above all, staff must be thoroughly trained and familiar with procedures to ensure the pre-admitted patient is given VIP treatment and processed quickly through the admitting area. When a patient presents for admission, they are asked immediately if they were pre-admitted. If so, they are taken immediately before all other patients. Nothing will destroy a pre-admission program quicker than unprepared staff, particularly if a physician finds out that his pre-admitted patient was delayed.

2

Inpatient Registration

Definitions

Registration—obtaining and recording demographic, financial and personal information for use by the hospital and other authorized parties to conduct business, as well as maintain legal medical records according to all applicable state and federal statutes.

Deposit—the estimated portion of the patient's bill not covered by insurance and paid or financed prior to or at the time of registration or discharge.

Inpatient—a registration requiring overnight service (with the exception of 23-hour observation patients).

Inpatient Registration

The recommended procedure for registering the direct admit patient is essentially the same as the procedure outlined in the pre-registration section. The primary difference is TIMING. In the case of a direct admit, the Registrar does not have the opportunity to double check information before the patient is registered, so it is imperative that each step of the registration process be followed in the proper sequence. Adherence to the following procedures will ensure the registration is handled properly.

Greeting the Patient

When the patient arrives at the hospital, the Registrar greets the patient, has the patient sign in, and requests insurance cards and driver's license. Once the patient is comfortable, the reservation book or log is checked to determine if a pre-admission was made.

Registration

The admitting and registration process should be very thorough with the primary goal being to get complete and accurate information while maintaining a very high public relations profile. This can be done as expeditiously as possible, subjecting the patient to as few forms as possible from the registration area.

Any form not involving what is necessary to complete the actual admitting process is the responsibility of the area requiring the forms.

The process is initiated by the patient's physician and completed by the hospital's registration department. Medical records *suspension lists* are checked at this time to ascertain whether the physician is eligible to admit patients (see policy Admitting Patients of Suspended Physicians). If physicians have been delinquent in completing patient charts in the past, their names will appear on this list. Hospital administration is then consulted for instructions on how to proceed. After accurately recording the physician's request for registration, the Registrar proceeds with the following:

- Complete the inpatient registration record
- Obtain signature for responsibility of hospital charges
- Obtain verification of legal age
- Check valuables
- Verify insurance coverage
- Settle self-pay estimate

An admitting checklist is thoroughly and accurately completed for each admission and filed in the patient's financial folder.

Completing the Registration Form

Include the following information on all registration forms:

Patient Information

- Full Name
- Full Address (include zip code)
- Telephone Number
- Date of Birth
- Gender
- Marital Status
- Next of Kin (not living with the patient) name, address, telephone number, relationship to patient
- Religion
- National Origin

Employment

- Employer
- Address
- Position
- Telephone Number
- Name of person handling group insurance
- Position
- Number of years employed

Spouse Information (if applicable)

- Name
- Address
- Employment information

Guarantor Information

- Full Name
- Address
- Telephone Number (residence)
- Employer (and telephone number)
- Position

Insurance Coverage

- All coverage applicable noted
- Medicare: H.I.B. number—PRO pre-admission approval is reviewed before proceeding
- Medicaid: identification number and current proof of eligibility
- Individual insurance policy: policy number, insurance company name and address, name of insured
- Group insurance: employer's name, address and telephone number, group number, insurance company name and address
- Blue Cross individual insurance: employer's name, address and telephone number, member's name, group number, certification number, coverage code
- Claimant's statement, if applicable
- Pre-authorization number, if applicable
- Special requirements, i.e., concurrent review, second surgical opinion, if applicable
- Mailing address for claims

Medical Information

- Name of attending physician
- Admitting diagnosis
- Medical necessity for private room accommodation should be documented and reported to DRG coordinator to check for documentation in physician's notes (Medicare only)
- Date and time of registration
- Classify as emergency, urgent, or elective

Accommodation Desired

- Private/semi-private/nursery
- Non-smoking/smoking

Previous Registration

- Inpatient or outpatient
- Name used
- Any member of immediate family

Patient or Guarantor Identification

- Driver's license
- Social security number
- Credit cards

Medicare patients must have an MSP screening form completed and signed. This form is placed in the patient's financial folder for billing purposes.

Medicare patients are given the form entitled "An Important Message from Medicare" at the time of admission.

History files should be checked for bad debts.

Signature on Conditions of Admission Form

All patients or guarantors must sign a "Conditions of Admission" form regardless of the type of coverage. This form indicates the intention to meet the hospital obligations should their insurance not be approved. In addition, it includes important responsibility information concerning valuables, nursing care, consent for treatment, release of information, and assignment of benefits.

If the patient is incompetent or unable to sign due to condition or age, the responsible party signs. Witnesses should be included when possible.

Determination of Financial Requirements

After completing the registration process, it is necessary to determine the financial requirements of the patient. The first step in this procedure is to verify third party coverage. **The third party carrier or employer should be called to verify coverage while the patient is in the registration office.**

The patient's estimated length of stay and anticipated charges should be determined. Additionally, the current account listings and bad debt listings are checked to determine if the patient owes a previous balance. The patient's required deposit can be calculated using a variable deposit policy. Copies should be made of insurance cards, Medicare cards, Medicaid cards, etc., and kept with the patient's financial file in the business office.

Communication of Financial Requirements

The patient or responsible party is requested to pay the deposit at the time of registration. If the deposit cannot be paid in full, other available deposit options are discussed—credit cards, payment arrangements—and referred to the Director of Admissions as appropriate, so a mutually satisfactory arrangement can be made. For after-hours and weekend admissions, a deposit is collected until insurance verification can be done. If the patient is unable to make a deposit, the manager-on-call is contacted for approval.

Situations involving patients having less than 100 percent coverage, and making no deposit, should be referred to the manager-on-call, Director of Admissions, or Business Office Manager. The manager notifies the physician of the patient's financial situation and asks if the registration can be transferred to a registered facility with funds to cover non-paying patient care. If the physician states that the registration can be rescheduled or the patient registered to another facility, the Director of Admissions or Business Office Manager notifies the patient to report back to the physician. All conversations with the patient and the physician are fully documented in the patient's financial file.

If the physician states that the patient is in need of immediate medical treatment, the patient must be registered without delay.

In this situation, the registration approval form is completed and immediately forwarded to the Business Office Manager, Chief Financial Officer, and Administrator with documentation of the conversation with the physician. The form is to be signed and dated by the individual approving the admission.

Patients presenting without third party payor identification are considered self-pay until valid proof of coverage is obtained.

Verification of Legal Age

If the patient has reached legal age, is married, or is an emancipated minor, permission for registration and treatment must be signed by the patient. If the patient is a legal minor, the Registrar should determine that the accompanying person is the natural parent or legal guardian. If so, the parent signs for permission and indicates relationship to the patient. If the minor's parents are not locally situated, the Registrar places a call to the patient's parents; the call is monitored by the nursing supervisor or the switchboard operator on an extension line. The Registrar identifies him or herself and the hospital, relates the situation and asks the parent's permission for the registration and treatment of their child. If permission is granted, the Registrar and party on the extension will witness that it was given. The parent is asked to follow up the verbal permission with a telegram. In some states, laws permit minors to give legal consent to certain types of treatment without notifying their parents, as is often the case with abortion. These laws, however, do not make the minor financially liable in most cases. The hospital attorney should be consulted before accepting a minor's signature for financial obligation.

If the patient is incompetent, or unable to sign and give permission for registration and treatment due to condition, the next of kin should sign. In cases of dire emergency where next of kin are not present, the attending physician should indicate that, in his or her qualified professional opinion, the registration is imperative. The opinion should be documented on the medical and financial record.

Valuables

Procedures for handling patient possessions during the registration process:

- Inquire if the patient brought any valuables to the hospital (e.g., watches, rings, money, dentures).
- Advise the patient that hospital policy limits hospital liability for any possessions taken to the room.
- Suggest that the patient send any valuables home with relatives.
- Offer to check all valuables for safekeeping in the safe.
- If the patient wishes to have the valuables checked, the Registrar should list each item separately. This information is recorded on a valuables receipt form, jewelry identified by color and shape, not disclosing type of stone or metal. The envelope could be designed to provide the patient with an itemized copy of the valuables deposited.

The patient and Registrar both sign the form.

- The patient's valuables, along with a copy of the valuables receipt, is then placed in a sealed container and given to an authorized person to place in the safe. Both the person opening the safe and the Registrar witness the placement of the valuables in the safe.
- An itemized copy of the valuables receipt is given to the patient with a copy of the form placed inside the envelope.
- Two hospital employees witness the opening of the valuables envelope on discharge or patient requests.
- After discharge, if valuables remain unclaimed for more than 90 days and at least two attempts have been made to contact the owner, the hospital's attorney is consulted regarding the state laws pertaining to disposition.

Patient Identification and Room Assignment

Once registration and financial arrangements are completed, the Registrar provides the patient with an identification bracelet, and assigns the patient to a room.

A patient should never be taken to a room without an identification bracelet.

The admitting staff maintains a room control board (bed board) to ensure accurate assignments. The board indicates which rooms and beds are occupied. To further facilitate placing patients properly and keeping informed of their location, a name and diagnosis system can be used.

Example:	Female patients	pink strip
	Male patients	blue strip
	Pediatric	white strip

The Registrar notifies the hospital switchboard and information desk of room assignments as soon as possible to enable the physician and relatives to contact the patient without delay.

Escort Patient to Room

Once registration is completed, the Registrar calls and informs the charge nurse of the admission. When the escort arrives for the patient, the Registrar provides room assignment information (if assigned by Admitting) and the medical chart. Admitting office personnel do not perform the escort function. The Registrar gives the quality assurance questionnaires (if utilized by the facility) to the patient at this time, and advises the patient how to complete the form.

Post-registration Procedures

After registration is complete and the patient is en route to the room, the Registrar performs the following steps:

- Places all documents in proper order in the financial file. (Establish a set order for filing these forms.)
- Sends copies of registration records as required (to lab, admitting physician, etc.).
- Ensures that the correct revenue source code and all other financial billing and marketing codes available are documented and properly keypunched (if the facility has on-line admitting).
- Places financial file in "in-house patients" file.
- Completes the registration log.

Registration Policies

Written registration policies must be approved by administration and strictly enforced. These policies include, but are not limited to, the following:

Discrimination

No hospital may discriminate in its registration policies or procedures with regard to race, age, religion, sex, color, or national origin at any time. *There are no exceptions.*

Financial Requirements

All financial requirements are enforced uniformly without regard to race, sex, color, religion, age, or national origin. Financial requirements, however, may vary depending on the nature, type, amount, reliability, or third party coverage. Hospitals reserve the right to ask for payments in full from any patient deemed not to have third party coverage sufficient or proven reliable enough to satisfy their financial obligation.

Charges for Services

Charges for services are applied uniformly to all patients. Gross charges are applied to all patient accounts without regard to types of coverage, ability to pay or length of stay.

Registration Deposits

Hospital policy provides for the verification of any third party coverage, estimation of length of stay based on admitting diagnosis and anticipated surgical procedures, computation of any self-pay amounts, and payment of these amounts either prior to or during the registration process. Exceptions to this policy, in the case of elective registration, should only be made by hospital administration and documented in the patient's financial files.

Third Party Coverage

Hospital policy states the hospital will, as a matter of courtesy and convenience to its patients, accept recognized third party coverage. Claims will be filed by the hospital for this coverage and the hospital will wait 30 days from the date of billing for payment. If, for any reason, payment is not made by the carrier, the hospital expects the balance to be paid in full by the patient. This policy should be explained to each patient at the time of registration and again at the time of discharge.

Hospital policies must be communicated to the patient prior to completion of the registration.

3

Emergency Room and Outpatient Registration

Definitions

Outpatient—is an individual receiving hospital-based or coordinated medical services for which the hospital is responsible. The outpatient does not require overnight service, with the exception of 23-hour observation patients.

Diagnostic Outpatient—is referred by a physician to a diagnostic or therapeutic facility for diagnosis or treatment on an ambulatory basis.

Emergency Outpatient—is registered to the emergency department, accident, or equivalent service of a hospital, requiring immediate diagnosis and treatment.

Same Day Surgery—patient receives surgical services as a diagnostic outpatient.

Recurring or Series Outpatient—is one for whom a definite and repeated treatment program is established for an extended period of time.

23-Hour Observation—is an expansion of the hospital's outpatient service to allow for evaluation, observation and implementation of treatment of patients with a medical need that may or may not require acute hospitalization. Patients may be held in the outpatient observation status for up to 23 hours and 59 minutes.

Introduction to Emergency Room and Outpatient Procedures

Utilization of hospital-based services by outpatients has significantly increased in recent years due to a number of factors. Since the cost of hospitalization is rising faster than many insurance coverages, patients frequently obtain diagnostic procedures on an outpatient basis instead of an inpatient basis. Furthermore, an increasing number of insurance companies are providing payment for diagnostic services not previously covered on an outpatient basis.

The volume of outpatient and emergency room procedures that generally occurs 24 hours a day, 365 days a year, necessitates clear, concise, and consistent written policies and procedures for the following activities:

- Establishing financial policies
- Controlling accounts receivable
- Registration process and systems
- Systems for monitoring effectiveness

The emergency room and outpatient staff should work within the framework of established policies. This ensures optimum treatment of patients and aids in the maintenance of financial management as well as physician and guest relations. Written emergency room and outpatient policies also facilitate the orientation and training of new employees. Failure to put all emergency room and outpatient policies in writing may result in:

- Inconsistent policies that foster criticism of the hospital
- Incorrect interpretation of policies by emergency room and outpatient registration personnel
- Misunderstanding by the medical staff or other hospital personnel about emergency room and outpatient policies
- Burdening administration with the necessity of making routine decisions
- Violation of legal requirements

- Increasing the total amount of time spent on processing an account
- Jeopardizing the financial operations of the hospital

The nature of the service a medical facility provides disallows denial of treatment.

Each outpatient and emergency room patient must receive treatment, if required by the physician.

It is therefore important to require adherence to financial policies.

Financial Policies

Post the hospital's financial policy in emergency and outpatient treatment areas.

Collect all monies due the hospital at the time of treatment.

Insurance is accepted for charges over an established minimum amount when acceptable insurance identification is provided. All patients who do not have acceptable insurance identification specifying their outpatient and emergency room coverage are expected to pay for services rendered. All outpatient and emergency room charges less than the minimum amount require cash payment of all charges, regardless of insurance coverage.

Acceptable insurance identification is a card, insurance policy, or telephone verification that the patient or responsible party has coverage for the services being rendered. Telephone verification is required if the card or policy does not specify the exact insurance coverage for the outpatient or emergency room services. If this is impossible, collection procedures should be initiated at the time of service. It is strongly suggested that telephone verification be obtained for all types of insurance coverage, regardless of the information stated on the card or policy.

Whether or not the patient pays in full, record the insurance information on the emergency room or outpatient chart. Insurance classifications acceptable in lieu of cash payment according to the guidelines stated above are:

- *Medicare:* Should be accepted for all services with acceptable identification card. The Registrar may ask patients if their Medicare Part "B" deductibles have been satisfied. If they have not, attempt to collect for the services rendered. The co-insurance should be requested for all services except clinical lab tests.
- *Medicaid:* Acceptable if recipients have *current* and valid identification cards or labels. If patients do not have cards, they should be asked to provide their caseworkers' names and be treated on a self-pay basis. (The term Medicaid is used to indicate all types of state funded welfare programs, although some states use the term Medical Assistance, and California uses the term Medi-Cal.)
- *Blue Cross and Blue Shield*
  Out-of-state: A collection effort should be made on all patients having out-of-state Blue Cross contracts.
- *Blue Cross and Blue Shield*
  In-state: Should be accepted if the patient has valid and acceptable identification card that specifies the insurance coverage for the services being rendered. Review the Blue Cross or Blue Shield manual for benefits. Benefits must be verified through Blue Cross.
- *Worker's Compensation:* Accept for all services based on proper verification that injury was a result of the patient's employment. Proper verification consists of written or verbal authorization for treatment by the patient's employer and worker's compensation carrier.
- *Personal Insurance:* Should be accepted if the patient has an acceptable identification card specifying coverage for the services being rendered. If not, collection should be made for the services rendered.
- *HMO/PPO:* Should be accepted if the HMO/PPO is listed as an approved contract and the necessary deductible or co-insurance collected as shown on the list of approved contracts. Verification should be made to the insurance carrier for an authorization number, when required.
- *Champus:* Should be accepted if the patient has a valid dependent's identification card. If patients live within 40 miles of a military medical facility, they must have a non-availability form.

Patients in all other classifications should be asked to pay for the balance owed at the time of service.

Patients and responsible parties must be informed, at the time of registration, of the hospital's outpatient and emergency room financial policies.

The hospital must enforce the financial policies and procedures fairly and consistently; however, policies should not cause undue hardship or create arguments with the patient, responsible party, or physician.

Under no circumstances should patients requesting emergency service be refused due to their inability to meet the financial requirements of the hospital.

Emergency Room and Outpatient Registration

The emergency and outpatient services provided by the hospital can only be effective if well-designed procedures are consistently enforced. Unlike other areas in the business office, the timing of necessary procedures cannot be controlled. Often, personnel handling emergency and outpatient services face situations demanding quick and accurate responses, making the registration process particularly challenging. By adhering to the following guidelines, however, the professional business office staff can be successful.

When the patient arrives, the Registrar proceeds with the following process:

- Greeting the patient
- Notification of physician and/or nursing personnel
- Registration
- Determination of financial requirements
- Communication of financial requirements
- Escort patient to the appropriate service areas

Greeting the Patient

The important first step in the process will vary depending on the type of patient. In every case, however, registration personnel endeavor to accommodate the patient. In a true emergency situation, medical attention is always the highest priority. Once the emergency room patient is being treated, the registration personnel obtain necessary information from the next of kin or other available sources. The exact procedure for registering an emergency room patient depends on whether the patient is a true emergency patient or diagnostic outpatient.

Notification of Physician or Nursing Personnel

Registration personnel should have an established procedure for all patients. For example, all ambulance (stretcher) patients must be seen immediately by an R.N.

> **The emergency room Registrar should never attempt triage of a patient unless the Registrar is duly qualified to do so.**

Registration

The need for accurate comprehensive information gathering is equally important for emergency room and outpatient registration as for inpatient. The major duties of the registration clerk are collecting cash and obtaining accurate patient information. Frequently, some medical information is also recorded during this process.

The major items of information to be recorded by the registration staff and medical personnel are as follows:

Patient Information

- Full Name
- Full Address (include zip code)
- Telephone Number
- Date of birth
- Gender
- Marital Status
- Next of Kin (not living with patient) name, address, telephone number, relationship to patient

Employer

- Name
- Address
- Position
- Telephone number
- Name of person handling group insurance
- Number of years on the job

Spouse Information, if Applicable

- Name
- Address
- Employment information

Guarantor Information

- Full name
- Address
- Telephone number
- Employer

Medical Information

- Name of attending physician and provider number
- Chief complaint and/or diagnosis
- Date and time of registration
- Emergency or non-emergency

Other Patient and Guarantor Information

- Copy of insurance card
- Driver's license
- Social security number
- Credit cards

Signatures

The registration staff is responsible for seeing that the necessary signatures of patient or responsible parties are gathered for the following:

- Assignment of insurance benefits (signed by policyholder)
- Financial responsibility
- Claimant's statement, as applicable
- Consent for treatment
- Authorization for the release of medical information
- Deposit of valuables
- Telephone consent, if the patient is a minor

Consent for treatment must be signed by the patient for any procedure performed within the hospital. This would apply to emergency room patients as well as diagnostic patients.

If the patient requires immediate treatment, only a limited amount of information can be obtained before the patient enters the treatment room:

- Patient's name and address
- Age and date of birth
- Gender
- Time and date of registration
- Patient's family physician
- Chief complaint

Previous Registrations and Visits

The active accounts receivable trial balance and bad debt listing are reviewed to determine if there are any previous outstanding bills or bad debts for either the patient or other family member. If unpaid bills exist, collect the outstanding amount in addition to the amount due for current services rendered.

Determination of Financial Requirements

As with inpatients, verify insurance coverage and collect any anticipated non-covered portions.

Itemized Charges Based on Requested Services and Procedure (Outpatient)

- Disposition: cash payment terms according to hospital policy
- Return: after treatment as necessary
- Telephone: follow up with ancillary departments
- Referrals: to other departments
- Return: to referring physicians

Communication of Financial Requirements

Once necessary registration information has been obtained and determination made whether the patient owes for any portion of the treatment, the patient (or guarantor) is advised of the amount due.

(The patient should be advised of this amount prior to treatment.)

When payment is requested, the patient is advised that credit cards are acceptable as well as cash and checks. Credit cards accepted by the hospital are displayed at the registration desk.

The terminology used in requesting payment from the patient can help determine whether or not the patient pays for his or her treatment. Following are examples of communicating charges:

Undesirable: "The charge is $75," or "The bill will be $75."

Desirable: "We estimate your portion of the bill to be $ _____ . Would you like to pay by cash, check, or credit card?"

Escort Patients to the Appropriate Service Areas

Patients may be directed to treatment areas. In emergency areas (and for stretcher and wheelchair patients), nursing personnel, volunteers, or other appropriate staff should escort patients. Emergency room and outpatient Registrars are not to leave their areas for this purpose. Ancillary departments should escort patients to the registration area when services are complete.

Routine Referred Outpatient Registration

Routine outpatient procedures are performed on a referral basis from the patient's private physician. These procedures are non-emergency in nature.

The patient is referred to the registration clerk along with written orders from the physician for the services to be performed.

The registration clerk obtains the patient's demographic and financial information as well as consent for treatment, authorization for release of information, insurance assignment, financial responsibility, and insurance claimant statement, if applicable.

Payment in full is collected for the scheduled procedure at the time of service, or proper insurance verification will be accepted and any required deposit collected. Exceptions to the financial policies may be made and documented only by the Business Office Manager, Chief Financial Officer, and/or Administrator.

The registration clerk retains a copy of the outpatient registration record. The remaining copies and requisitions are sent to the appropriate ancillary departments with the patient.

The Business Office Manager or appropriate person must always contact the physician before canceling procedures due to financial reasons.

All patients are registered through the business office registration department and not in separate ancillary areas. Ancillary departments should never perform tests prior to registration.

Same Day Surgery Registration

The registration personnel are assigned work hours from 7:00 A.M. to 3:00 P.M., Monday through Friday, or according to surgery times and volume of patients.

The physician schedules operating time with the operating room and/or admitting at least three days in advance of the scheduled surgery. At this time, the surgeon provides operating room personnel with the physician's orders, and registration personnel with patient information.

The physician notifies the patient that a pre-surgical appointment will be necessary. At the same time, the physician advises the patient that payment in full, acceptable insurance information, or a combination is required prior to surgery. (Any questions are clarified by the pre-admission clerk through the routine pre-admission process.)

Written treatment orders are preferred, though not required, since orders may be called in to the operating room (O.R.) scheduling staff. Written instructions must follow telephone orders, prior to surgery.

A conference call between the physician, registration, and O.R. scheduling staff saves time since the physician's office is only required to make one call and all available information can be relayed simultaneously.

The operating room personnel provide the outpatient registration personnel with a surgery schedule prior to each day's surgery, calling immediately with late additions. The registration personnel telephone the patient confirming the date and time of surgery and arrange a pre-surgical appointment time. The patient is informed of the approximate charges and the hospital's financial policies regarding payment prior to services rendered.

In the event patients arrive for surgery and admitting was not notified, or if a list of surgeries is not received daily, the Business Office Manager is advised.

The same day surgery chart is created at the pre-surgical appointment, if not in advance.

Consent for surgery form is completed when the patient is registered.

Insurance assignment of benefits, financial responsibility, claimant's statement if applicable, consent for treatment, and release of medical information forms are completed and signed when the patient is registered.

Copies of insurance information are made.

Insurance coverage and benefits must be verified prior to rendering service.

Department requisition slips are embossed with the patient charge plate or on-line entry performed.

The registration clerk presents a pre-operative instruction sheet and financial policy to the patient.

The patient is instructed to report to the registration clerk approximately two hours prior to the scheduled surgery time.

When the patient arrives on the day of surgery, the registration clerk is responsible for the following:

- Collecting payment or insurance information for the scheduled procedure based on the financial policies.
- Notifying operating room personnel that the registration is complete.
- Calling to have the patient transported to the operating room unit.

Upon discharge, the patient is escorted by nursing service back to the registration clerk for collection of charges, documentation, and filing of the patient folder.

The scheduled same day surgery procedures are subject to cancellation if financial requirements cannot be met. The Business Office Manager must contact the attending physician prior to notifying the patient of the cancellation.

Recurring or Series Outpatient Registration

This category includes patients who have been scheduled by their physician to be treated at the hospital intermittently for an extended period of time (weeks or months). A common example of this is recurring physical therapy.

It is important to control recurring patients from a financial perspective. The recommended procedure involves the use of 3 × 5 cards to accommodate a manual control system for hospitals whose computer systems are not sophisticated enough to effectively manage the account.

Patients who are going to have more than one visit per month may be set up as recurring accounts.

All recurring account patients have 3 × 5 cards made with the patient name, number, and date of registration. The cards are filed alphabetically in a card file.

The computer is profiled, if possible, to automatically discharge any recurring account patients who have not received any charges for thirty days.

When bills are generated by the system, any recurring account bill that has been discharged should have the corresponding 3 × 5 card pulled and thrown away.

This method will control the recurring account patients. When each patient arrives, the 3 × 5 file is checked for a recurring account card. The account number and patient name are written on a charge ticket and given to the patient to receive services. If the 3 × 5 card does not exist, the patient is not a recurring account and the patient will have to be registered as a new patient.

Ancillary departments should not treat anyone unless the patient has a charge ticket or other form with the account number.

Billing holds all recurring account files in a separate file alphabetically so they can be billed monthly. When the patient is discharged and final billed, the folder goes back to the central files.

If a patient, including nursing home patient, maintains as a recurring account patient for 90 days, the account is manually discharged and re-registered by asking the patient for all demographic information to obtain any updated information.

OB Observation Patients

The pre-admit patient number is used for services rendered in cases where an OB patient has been preadmitted and then is brought in for observation for a period of less than 24 hours. A new pre-admit packet is made for the return delivery and a new patient number assigned.

To achieve maximum results in the accounts receivable management program, controls must be put in place to ensure that all demographics are taken down accurately and completely, insurance is verified at the time of registration, deposits are requested, and financial arrangements are made prior to or at the time of registration.

II

Third Party Payors

4

Types of Third Party Payors and Billing Requirements

Definitions

Third Party—Insurance coverage that pays a portion (or all) of total charges on a patient account.

First Party—patient
Second Party—hospital
Third Party—insurance company/payor

Insurance Claim—The statement of total charges on patient accounts (standard form is the UB-82) that are examined by insurance companies to pay liability as stated in the terms of the policy (contract) between the patient and insurance company.

Insurance Coverage—The insurance payment liability on an insurance claim as stated in the terms of the policy (contract) between the patient and insurance company.

Timely Filing—The shortest time period (five days should be the goal) between hospital discharge and claim completion mailed or carried to the patient's insurance company.

UB-82—The standard insurance claim form issued for general use in 1984 to complete third party billing to all insurance carriers, although a limited few third parties and fiscal intermediaries still require their own forms.

Accounts Receivable Insurance Billing Plans

It is important for all billing personnel to be familiar with the various types of coverage. This section provides an overview of the most common plans encountered. Each plan is discussed in terms of its most important features.

Medicare—Title XVIII

Medicare is a federal program that pays for health care provided to eligible people 65 years of age or older and to qualified disabled individuals. Medicare is offered through the Social Security Administration of the Department of Health and Human Services (HHS). There are various fiscal intermediaries for hospitals in each state. A fiscal intermediary is a private insurance company that may administer the Medicare program (act as an agent) for Social Security Administration. A hospital may also contract directly with SSA in Baltimore.

Each hospital business office should have a copy of the *Medicare Hospital Manual* and make certain that changes are made as received from the fiscal intermediary. The fiscal intermediary also publishes periodic newsletters that provide additional billing instructions. These should be kept in a permanent file. Involved billing personnel are to be kept informed of its contents.

Medicare is a two-part program:

- *Part A*—Hospital Insurance for stay and treatment while in the hospital. This part pays hospital providers for services rendered to Medicare beneficiaries.
- *Part B*—Supplementary Medical Insurance. Part B pays for medically necessary physician services, outpatient services, home health care, and various medical services and supplies not covered by Part A. Hospitals must accept assignments for Medicare Part B coverage and accept the amounts paid. Part B charges disallowed by Health Care Financing Administration (HCFA) cannot be billed to the patient by the hospital; however, hospitals may bill 20

percent of the charges, minus any clinical lab charges, plus any remaining deductible to the patient. The *Medicare Hospital* and *Provider* manuals can be consulted for specific information concerning which hospital charges are covered.

Medicare deductibles:

- *Inpatient Deductible:* a predetermined amount payable by the patient annually.
- *Outpatient Deductible:* a predetermined amount payable by the patient once a year for outpatient services. This can also apply to physician billings. Once the outpatient deductible is satisfied for the year, no further deductible is due.

Information necessary for billing Medicare includes the following:

- Patient's name as it appears on the Medicare card.
- Patient's HIB number as it appears on the Medicare card.
- In most cases, letters after the social security number (suffix) represent the classification of a Medicare patient. Listed are the most common letters:

  A: A person who worked and made contributions to SSA for the required time period(s).

  B: A person who never contributed to SSA, but whose eligibility is determined by a spouse's contribution record.

  C: A child of a person dependent on someone who worked under SSA.

  D: A widow/widower of a person dependent on someone who worked under SSA.

  W: A disabled widow/widower under age 65 collects under the spouse's number if he/she was disabled prior to death.

  J: A person who turned 72 prior to 1968 and had not worked enough quarters under SSA, but was made eligible by a special Act of Congress.

  M: Generally denotes *medical benefits only.* If the patient has hospital benefits, the card will so state.

  T: An individual entitled to Part A benefits, but not to Retirement and Survivor's or Railroad Retirement Insurance, or who is entitled to Medicare based on chronic renal disease. It applies whether or not the beneficiary elects to receive Part B.

- Medicare numbers that have a prefix (a letter before the number) generally denote retired railroad employees who have Medicare.
- The above list is not all-inclusive. The letters listed simply represent the classifications most commonly applied to Medicare recipients.
- Hospitals should make a photocopy of the Medicare card for confirmation of classification.

SSA requires all fiscal intermediaries to accept Medicare claims on the UB-82 claim form (SSA-1450). **HCFA has required, effective January 1, 1986, that all claims be submitted electronically to avoid automatic 21-day delay in claims processing.**

Medicare billing requires a definitive final diagnosis, operative procedures with corresponding DRG code and ICD-9-CM codes as well as the DRG. HCPCS codes are required for outpatient clinical lab tests, radiology procedures and ambulatory surgical procedures.

- Diagnosis-Related Group (DRG): the DRG program is a hospital reimbursement method that pays a flat rate for a particular pre-defined diagnosis.
- ICD-9-CM, CPT-4 and HCPCS coding: numeric coding systems identified by diagnosis or procedure for reimbursement purposes.

Billings for physical therapy, cardiology and occupational therapy require therapist information.

Follow-ups on claims are directed to the fiscal intermediary.

The hospital notifies the patient in writing when registering for those services that are not covered by the Medicare program. This informs patients of their responsibility for these charges if the services are used. The hospital keeps patients notified that Medicare will not pay for certain services; otherwise, patients cannot be held responsible. Patients must sign this documentation as confirmation that they have been informed.

Medicaid—Title XIX

(Title XIX may be identified as Medicaid, Medical Assistance or other names in certain states, such as Medi-Cal in California. The term "Medicaid" will be used in this manual.)

Medicaid is a welfare program funded by state and federal agencies. It pays for health care service provided to persons qualified under the program. Medicaid is a state-administered program and each state decides whether it wants the program, what services it will provide, and to whom; however, Medicaid must cover certain welfare recipients, mothers who are on Aid to Dependent Children, children who are wards of the state (foster children), and provide items of basic medical care that are specified in the Social Security Act.

Information required for billing Medicaid includes the following:

- The Medicaid provider number must be entered on all claims.
- Sterilization consents and medical necessity for some admissions must be included with the claim. The Medicaid manual can be referred to for specific state requirements.
- When Medicaid recipients visit a hospital outside their home state, the out-of-state provider hospital confirms the policies applicable under the home state Medicaid plan. In many situations, the out-of-state hospital must fill out an application for provider status under the Medicaid home plan. Information regarding this application and the subsequent billing requirements may be obtained through the state's fiscal intermediary for Medicaid. To determine where to contact the fiscal intermediary, the out-of-state provider contacts the home state's department of human resources in the capital.
- Many Medicaid intermediaries offer programs for CRT, tape-to-tape, and electronic billing. Hospitals having the capability to participate in these programs can consult with their state's Medicaid fiscal intermediary.

Worker's Compensation

The purpose of worker's compensation is the provision of insurance coverage by employers for employees who are *injured* or *ill* as a result of their employment. All employees are covered except federal employees, agricultural employees, and domestic employees. This may vary from state to state.

It is important to note that although worker's compensation may represent a small segment of the total accounts receivable, there can be a delay in reimbursement. Follow-up will normally be on a case-by-case basis and should be initiated by first contacting the insurance carrier, then the patient's employer, the state Industrial Accident board, and ultimately, the patient.

Certain information is essential to the collection of payment regarding worker's compensation:

- Patient's full name and social security number
- Name of employer, including address and telephone number
- Name and address of employer's worker's compensation insurance company and policy/case number
- Date and time of accident (employer's report of injury, as applicable)
- Confirmation by employer of worker's compensation status

The physician is kept informed about coverage. Likewise, the physician should keep the hospital informed of any change in diagnosis or in the provision of services *not* associated with the job-related illness or injury.

It is important to understand the basic relationship that exists between the hospital and the patient's employer in a claim involving worker's compensation. The carrier is simply an intermediary, therefore, the employer must be listed as a responsible party when it authorizes treatment. The patient or guarantor must be listed as a responsible party of all treatment related to noncompensable injuries.

In addition, it should be noted that states have their own worker's compensation laws, and most state laws require carriers to pay only for reasonable charges in worker's compensation cases. In many states, a patient's failure to report injury within 24 hours can negate coverage.

It cannot be assumed that a patient is covered by worker's compensation. The hospital should always ask for additional coverage.

If a claim is denied (assuming it is not denied because of hospital oversight), the billing department is responsible for:

- Identifying additional coverage
- Contacting the patient for payment
- Contacting the employer (guarantor) for payment

The hospital is under no obligation to wait for appeal activity or legal action to recover damages.

Blue Cross

Blue Cross is a nonprofit organization covering hospital, medical, surgical, and major medical.

Some states have several Blue Cross associations representing regions of that state. Other states may have one association with a single central headquarters. Most Blue Cross inpatient claims must be submitted through the in-state Blue Cross Interplan Bank, which contacts the home plan for benefits when the patient has out-of-state plan coverage. Some Blue Cross inpatient claims must be submitted directly to the home plan for out-of-state claims.

This procedure varies from state to state. Out-of-state outpatient claims are usually billed directly to the out-of-state home plan.

Although the majority of Blue Cross members have membership through group coverage, individual policies are also provided. Blue Cross also provides supplementary coverage for Medicare beneficiaries.

Blue Cross provides member hospitals a *Provider Manual* that sets forth coverage and billing instructions concerning procedures for billing on the UB-82.

Information necessary for billing Blue Cross:

- Patient's full name
- Policyholder's full name
- Membership and certificate number
- Coverage code
- Group number
- Employer's name, address, and telephone number (if applicable)
- Final diagnosis and surgical procedures
- Pre-authorization number, when applicable

Make a copy of the membership card for confirmation of the above information and attach the copy to the Blue Cross billing.

Blue Cross may provide member hospitals with billing forms, depending on the association within the state; however, most associations use a standard UB-82 format.

Blue Cross requires primary and secondary diagnoses plus applicable operative procedure(s) that come from medical records ICD-9-CM (International Classification of Diseases—Clinical Modifications).

A copy of the itemized statement is filed with the claim.

The hospital must submit a Notice of Admission on the day of registration for verification of benefits in state associations that require this information.

Follow-up of the insurance payment with Blue Cross should occur regardless of individual or group coverage. If no change in payment status occurs, follow up with the employer and policyholder direct.

Generally, Blue Cross pays claims on a weekly basis.

Blue Cross representatives make periodic visits to assist with any problems that may arise. They are known as Provider Representatives.

Contractual conflicts can develop when there are two policies involved in coordination of benefits; they can be resolved by follow-up with both employers and carriers.

Several states now employ systems that will allow a hospital to use a CRT terminal to record patient ID and instantly verify coverage. Tape-to-tape billing arrangements already exist in some states and trial programs are underway in others. Each hospital should investigate these programs through its Blue Cross fiscal intermediaries.

Since Blue Cross is generally a nonprofit, cost-based health contract, provisions for regulation are usually covered separately under insurance codes. Hospital personnel should become familiar with the state insurance code provisions for Blue Cross in the respective state.

Champus

Champus is a benefit provided for dependents of military personnel. There are two kinds of Champus:

Active Champus: benefits—full coverage less deductible.

Retired Champus: benefits—75 percent coverage.

In order for an active Champus patient to use a private hospital, he must obtain a nonavailability form (DD1251). This assures the hospital that the procedure cannot be carried out at the base hospital and that Champus will pay the private facility. Military dependents who **do not** live within 40 miles of a military medical facility are not required to have a nonavailability form.

UB-82 is the claim form utilized for billing Champus beneficiaries.

A patient registered under Champus must have a valid dependent's ID card. Patients, if spouses of members of the military, must have their own cards. Children over ten years of age must have their own cards.

ChampVA

Similar to Champus, ChampVA requires the insured to be a disabled veteran's spouse, dependent, or survivor of those who died of service-connected causes. These patients do not need nonavailability forms. Both Campus and ChampVA use the same forms and these forms are completed using the patient's ID card.

Liability Cases

Liability cases must have administrative approval. Usually the attorney will call and assure the hospital protection of the bill, but this is not sufficient. The attorney should be asked for a letter of guarantee. This can simply be a letter from the attorney guaranteeing that the hospital will be paid out of any proceeds received. Most liabilities involve motorcycle or auto accidents. **It is recommended that a lien or notice of claim be filed to protect the hospital's interest.**

Liability claims typically involve lengthy lawsuits. Therefore, it is advisable to try to obtain any information on other coverage.

Commercial Insurance

Commercial insurance is available to cover most aspects of health care (hospital, medical, surgical, major medical, disability, mental health, and substance abuse).

Information required for billing commercial insurance:

- Patient's full name
- Full name of policyholder
- Membership number/policy number
- Group number (if applicable), employer's name, address, and telephone number
- Special billing instructions
- Final diagnosis (also surgical procedure)
- Payroll ID number
- Authorization for release of medical information

Obtain an assignment of benefits for payment directly to the hospital. The patient's refusal to assign benefits will mean that the account must be handled as self-pay and the necessary deposit collected.

Although UB-82 forms are available, some companies still require completion of special forms or claimant's statements in addition to the UB-82. The hospital should request that carriers or companies requiring claimant's statements supply the hospital with these forms so patients may complete the forms prior to discharge. Copies of claimant's statements are kept in the patient financial file and the original sent with the original claim.

A copy of the itemized statement must be filed with the claim.

Although most companies require that the physician's portion of the form be completed prior to payment, hospitals may submit a copy of the completed form to the insurance company or employer (in the case of group coverage) prior to submission by the physician. Such steps help to establish a claim for payment as early as possible.

Depending on the insurance policy, the hospital will follow up the payment of benefits directly with the insurance company, through the patient's employer, or with the patient.

Individual Insurance: Individual coverage is a policy purchased from an insurance company directly by the individual. Benefits payable under these plans usually do not coordinate with other coverages the individual may own. Some group plans may be converted to individual coverage after an employee leaves a company.

Group Insurance: Group coverage is insurance purchased through an employer or other organizational body where the individual and the group share the premium cost at an overall discount. Group policies coordinate benefits with other groups, yet not with individual plans.

Copies of all billing forms, including, but not limited to the UB-82, itemized statement, claimant's statement, assignment of benefits, copies of cards or other identification are kept in the patient financial file.

Health Maintenance Organizations

Health Maintenance Organizations (HMO's) vary in structure, form, and ideals. They operate on a provider cost basis, per diem basis, or charge basis. The billing system is worked out on an individual basis when a hospital becomes a provider for an HMO. HMO members are usually individuals or companies who pay a set monthly amount (in lieu of insurance coverage) and in turn are treated without additional cost. There may be a co-insurance or deductible amount, which is payable by the patient. HMO's contract with hospitals to provide care. Usually, charges to HMO's are discounted or provided on a contractual reduced price.

No Insurance

On self-pay bills, an itemized statement stamped "Insurance Assigned to Hospital" is sent to patients so the hospital will be notified if the patients file insurance claims on their own. After mailing the itemized statement, the account should be forwarded to the Collection Department.

State Plans

This type of coverage is usually designed to provide financial assistance for specialized treatment in areas related to crippled children, physical rehabilitation, and renal dialysis. Each state organization requires different information in administering such appropriations. Billing is usually documented on a state voucher form and directed to the state comptroller's office. Any questions concerning these types of programs should be directed to the state's department of health and human resources.

Charitable Organizations

Billings directed to charitable organizations for such disabilities and diseases as blindness and cancer should be discussed with the particular organization that will be providing funds.

Federal Plans

This coverage deals with group insurance for federal employees. The federal government contracts with private insurance companies as fiscal intermediaries to administer their programs. Appeals for non-payment of claims are made through the federal agency that sponsors the insurance coverage. Appeals are made by the policyholder directly to the agency. Billings are handled in the same manner as all other group insurance claims and are directed to the fiscal intermediary.

Worker's compensation for federal employees is handled by the U.S. Department of Labor. Responsibility for processing these claims is centralized in regional offices throughout the country. For information regarding the office that handles these claims in a particular area, contact the nearest U.S. Department of Labor office.

Union Plans

Although billed in the same manner as all other group plans, union plans are usually administered as self-insured programs; therefore, these plans are not governed by the state insurance commission.

Estate Cases

Claims are always filed against a deceased patient's estate. Contact the local probate court to determine if there is an estate and how to file a claim, regardless of third party coverage indicated on the patient's file.

UB-82 Billing Manual

The *UB-82 Billing Manual* contains detailed explanations of information necessary for billing claims to an insurance company. The manual was written for Medicare billing; therefore, some items that may be required for billing Medicare are not required for other insurance billings. Refer to the *UB–82 Billing Manual* for assistance in billing claims or establishing computer profiles.

Certified Mail Claims

Claims exceeding $1,000, excluding those electronically submitted, can be sent by certified mail, return receipt requested. This ensures that problem carriers cannot deny receipt of larger dollar amount claims.

5

Third Party Coverage Verification

A third party is an individual, group of individuals, or an organization that functions as an intermediary between the hospital and the patient by providing payment to the hospital for services rendered. Third party payors include Blue Cross, Medicare, Medicaid, state agencies, HMO's, commercial insurance, worker's compensation, Champus, self-insured employers and other charitable agencies. Payment by these third parties make up the major portion of the hospital's reimbursement of revenue. Although about 90 percent of patients requiring hospital care are covered by some form of insurance, many patients are unfamiliar with their coverage limits until hospitalization is required. The hospital should verify and interpret the patient's insurance coverage prior to or at the time of registration and should inform the patient. This will prepare the patient to face any financial obligation due to the limitation of coverage. The hospital can avoid instances involving insurance claims being rejected in whole or in part because of insufficient benefits by verifying coverage prior to registration.

As soon as the reservation form is completed, the preadmission clerk must verify the coverage available. Verification must always be included in the pre-registration process.

Calling for benefits is the most important step in the insurance verification process. The information obtained at this time forms the basis for all subsequent steps in the process.

To facilitate the verification process, and to verify benefits after hours and on weekends, establish an insurance verification master file. The master file allows verification to be completed by confirming an employee's participation in the insurance program with the employer. For after-hours registrations, the hospital will assume that the insurance is in force on presentation of an insurance card or evidence of employment until the employer can be contacted.

To begin an insurance verification master file, a letter and benefits form is sent to all employers within the hospital's service area requesting they forward the necessary insurance information, including contract renewal date, to the hospital. A master file index sheet is completed for each company responding. It includes the name and address of the insurance company; name, title, and telephone extension of the person providing information; and the contract renewal date. Once made, the card is filed in the master file. An index sheet is also prepared for any new information obtained.

Many types of insurance or health benefit plans are similar in structure, yet very few are alike in coverage limits, forms required, pre-existing conditions, coordination of benefits, eligibility, assignability, and other related standards. Each coverage type has unique elements specifically related to the policies' sponsors.

Hospital personnel performing verification should be able to obtain, interpret, and relay this information so the other business office departments may properly secure payment.

Pre-call Planning

Establishing pre-call standards for verification of insurance for registration will help the hospital avoid the pitfalls of not obtaining complete information.

Review available information from pre-registration/ registration records:

- Patient's name
- *Insured* party
- Name of the insurance carrier
- Kind of insurance (group, individual, government)
- Group policy number, certificate number, payroll number, etc.
- Is there a valid insurance assignment?
- Is it a work related injury?
- Is there more than one carrier?
- Who is the primary carrier?
- Claim form required?

Establish the call objectives. Determine patient eligibility for coverage and the insurance benefits covered.

Determine who will be called:

- Employer's personnel office
- Insurance carrier
- Insurance agent (third party liability)
- Union
- Charitable Organization
- State Agency Department

Review additional questions due to diagnosis type:

- Psychiatric
- Cosmetic Surgery
- Newborn
- Substance Abuse
- Rehabilitation

Making the Phone Call

Identify the caller and the hospital.

Give reason for the call, stating name of patient and name of the *insured*.

Confirm that caller is speaking to the proper person for verification of coverage and benefits.

Ask fact finding questions in relation to the insurance verification sheet:

- Is patient covered?
- How long has policy been in effect?
- Are there unpaid premiums or union dues?
- Does responsible party have sufficient employment hours?
- What are the basic benefits?
- What are the major medical benefits?
- What are the physician benefits?
- Is there a pre-existing condition clause?
- Is there a coordination of benefits clause?
- Are there other limitations due to diagnosis type, i.e., psychiatric, group or occupational therapy?
- What forms are necessary for billing? (For example, claimant's statement.)
- Where and to whom should the bill be sent?
- What portion of benefits have been used?
- Is concurrent review required?
- If this is a work related injury, what is the claim number?
- Is pre-authorization necessary? Number? Authorizing party's name?
- Is re-certification required? How many days authorized?

Request assistance in completing insurance verification form.

Confirm the name and title of the person who provided the information. Record the time of the call.

If the benefits verified are not present in the insurance verification master file, complete a master file index sheet and catalog appropriately.

Rarely will an insurance company guarantee payment on a patient account either verbally or in writing. Companies will verify the information listed in their records at the time a call is made. This is simply a relay of information and in no way obligates the insurance company to pay the hospital according to the benefits verbalized.

Payment assurances from third party payors may be obtained by using one of the following procedures:

- Send the confirmation of benefits verification form by mail.
- Advise the patient or employer to present a letter from the employer to this effect to certify that the injury is work related at the time of admission. (It is important to verify employment and length of service when the patient is a compensation case or covered by a group insurance plan related to employment, or even self-pay.)

In worker's compensation cases, verify that a report of injury has been submitted by the employer and received by the insurance carrier or agent.

To complete the verification process, check thoroughly:

- Verification form has all applicable items completed to ensure proper billing information.
- This information is legible and correct.
- All benefit information is comprehensive and includes basic major medical and physician benefits.
- The full name, location, and title of the person(s) from whom verification is documented on the verification form.

At the time insurance is verified, a file card is prepared with the name and address of the insurance company and the name, title, and telephone extension of the person providing information, if the insurance is not listed in the Master Insurance Index. *Building coverage reference (Master Insurance Index) files will prove invaluable for future verification.* Once verification is completed, all files are returned to the in-house patient financial file location.

Birthday Rule: When a child is treated and there is double coverage from both parents, the primary carrier is determined by the birthday rule. The parent with the earliest birth month of the year is the primary policyholder. The other policy will usually coordinate benefits to cover any deductible or co-insurance from the first payor.

Troubleshooting Verification Problems

The following chart discusses the most common problems encountered during the insurance verification process, and provides corresponding solutions.

After Hours Verification

Common Cause	Recommended Solution(s)
Most insurance companies do not offer 24-hour verification of insurance. Even companies with CRT computer communication are "down" during certain times of the day or night for update and maintenance.	• Develop an insurance verification master file catalogued by employer that will list and define coverage contract date. • Require that the insured party or patient produce evidence of employment (I.D. badge, payroll check stub, insurance card) that will provide an indication of coverage. • Require the patient to submit a *hold check* for total estimated charges to the hospital in lieu of verification. Explain to the patient that the check will be returned if the insurance is verified at 100 percent and may be deposited if the insurance covers less than 100 percent of total charges.

Employer Verifies, Insurance Company Denies

Common Cause	Recommended Solution(s)
Occasionally, the employer verifies the patient's or insured's employment and eligibility for insurance coverage, but the insurance company has no record of this person.	• Re-contact the employer and explain the situation. Ask the employer to call the insurance company so that complete verification may be obtained. Indicate that a follow-up call will be placed in the next hour to determine if the situation has been resolved. • If the patient must be registered and the verification parties cannot be reached or if the situation cannot be resolved within the designated time period, request that the patient submit a *hold check* for total estimated charges. • Generally, the employer is the primary verification party in this instance. These situations are usually caused by a communication delay between employer and the insurance company, unpaid premiums, and misunderstanding of benefits.

Insurance Agent Verifies, Insurance Company Denies

Common Cause	Recommended Solution(s)
Many individuals purchase private insurance policies from independent insurance agents or brokers. Different arrangements are made for different people. Unfortunately, in this situation, there is no single, reliable verification source.	• Verification is not complete until a written guarantee of payment is submitted to the hospital either by the agent/broker or the insurance company.

Employer Lack of Knowledge

Common Cause	Recommended Solution(s)
Some employers will contract with an insurance company to totally administer a group insurance program for their company. In these cases, the employer will have little if any information about the coverage plan.	• Verification is not complete until the insurance carrier commits total eligibility and coverage verification.

Unpaid Union Dues or Premiums

Common Cause	Recommended Solution(s)
Insurance coverage for an individual may lapse due to unpaid premiums or union dues.	• Registration with this prospective coverage is not considered until written verification (indicating the covered time period until the next premium is due) is obtained from the insurance company.

Exhausted Benefits

Common Cause	Recommended Solution(s)
On all group and individual verifications, coverage and benefit limitations were not compared with confirmation of previous claims submitted within the patient's benefit period.	• If the patient's benefits are verified as exhausted, the patient must be informed that the registration will be handled on a self-pay basis.

Non-assignable Policies

Common Cause	Recommended Solution(s)
Non-assignable insurance coverage occurs when the insurance company is obligated by policy or contract agreement to always pay the patient directly for reimbursement of medical treatment. Consequently, the hospital cannot be paid directly from the insurance company and must depend on the patient to forward the payment received from the insurance company.	• Patients should be informed about the non-assignable provision of their insurance coverage. The insurance should not be accepted by the hospital and the registration should be handled on a self-pay basis.

Allocated Insurance Benefits

Common Cause	Recommended Solution(s)
Many individual policies offer allocated benefits that provide a specific benefit for each type of treatment that may be rendered. Insurance companies are generally reluctant to list the numerous reimbursement allocations to the hospital.	• Exercise extreme caution when considering these policies as valid coverage. These policies can be risky.

Resolution of problems encountered at the time of verification may make the difference between a collectable receivable or a bad debt.

Verifiable and Unverifiable Insurance Coverage and Benefits

Unverifiable

Insurance card without effective date or expiration date.

Insurance card with effective and expiration dates when verified employment dates do not concur.

Insurance cards for individual policies from certain companies without home office verification. These insurance companies provide a daily benefit indemnity plan that is usually payable directly to the patient. Temporary cards are sent to *prospective clients* prior to actual purchase or agreement. These temporary cards may be presented to the hospital as valid insurance coverage. The back of the card must be read completely; coverage cannot be assumed.

Payroll check stubs *may not* be used to verify benefits.

Employees of the same company where the patient works, other than the administrative or personnel departments.

Verbal authorization from employee supervisors for worker's compensation treatment.

Verbal authorization for treatment by attorneys.

Verbal authorization for treatment from insurance agents. (This type of verification must be guaranteed in writing.)

Verbal authorization for treatment in liability cases, including hotels, motels, amusement parks, department stores, or auto accidents. (Written guarantees of payment must be submitted for verification of these coverage types.)

Medicaid authorization letters in lieu of computerized cards, unless the patient's number is listed on the department's official records. (The state's department of human resources or social services can be contacted.)

Copies of policies with no dates. (Premiums may be unpaid.)

Verifiable

Patient's individual insurance carrier.

Patient's employer's personnel department.

Written guarantee of payment from patient's insurance agent or broker.

Written guarantee of payment from entity at fault in a liability case.

Voucher from the state to render treatment on sponsored patient.

Claims adjustor for employer's worker's compensation carrier.

Copy of insurance policy reflecting effective and expiration dates and showing premiums paid in full.

Insurance card reflecting effective and expiration dates as the verified employment dates concur.

Helpful Hints

Insurance Verification

Coverage Type	Establish Verification and Check
Medicare	• U.R. or Admitting Nurse's approval to admit • Copy of Medicare card • Both Part A and Part B are included in the patient's coverage • Deductible and co-insurance are collected • Any other supplemental insurance to cover deductible and co-insurance amounts • If hospitalization is required as a result of an auto accident or other liability in which liability coverage precedes Medicare coverage • Same diagnosis re-admit within 30 days

Helpful Hints—*Continued*

Coverage Type	Establish Verification and Check
Medicaid	• U.R. or Admitting Nurse's approval to admit • Copy of card • Refer to Medicaid manual for rules and regulations
Worker's Compensation	• Date of injury • Verification from employer that the report of injury has been filed and that coverage is authorized • Confirmation from the compensation carrier that the report of injury, if applicable, has been received and treatment may be rendered for the specified injury • Ensure only treatment for the specified injury will be rendered • Social security number—full patient name • Full name and address of compensation claims adjustor and employer

The hospital must never assume that a patient is covered by worker's compensation. Registrars must always ask for additional coverage and an assignment taken in case unrelated treatment is given.

Coverage Type	Establish Verification and Check
Blue Cross	• Copy of card • Notice of admissions (N.O.A.) sent, if required • Certificate number, group number, coverage code if applicable • Employer • Dependent coverage • Pre-existing clause • Effective date of policy • Cancel or expiration date of policy • Pre-authorization number

Helpful Hints—*Continued*

Coverage Type	Establish Verification and Check
Champus	• Copy of Champus I.D. card (both sides) • Expiration and effective dates • DD1251 or non-availability statement (if the residence is within a 40-mile radius of a military medical facility) and registration is non-emergent • Privacy Act form is signed and the patient's information is completed by the beneficiary and kept on file • The physician has signed the form certifying emergency status on emergent registrations • Determine whether Champus sponsor is active duty or retired • If patients are 10 years or over, they must have their own I.D. cards • If patients are over 18 years of age, they must sign the insurance form

Champus requires patients to certify any other coverage they may have on registration to the hospital.

ChampVA	• See Champus • All ChampVA benefits are concurrent with retired Champus; there is no need for a DD1251
Liability Insurance	• Letter of guarantee or cash • Other insurance coverage • Date, time, and location of accident • Approval by administration • Name of patient's attorney (if applicable)

The hospital cannot assume that a patient will be covered by liability coverage or take verbal authorization. Letters of guarantee along with a completed lien form are required as well as assignment on other insurance for treatment of non-related injuries or conditions.

Helpful Hints—*Continued*

Coverage Type	Establish Verification and Check
Commercial Group Insurance	• Copy of card • Full name of policyholder and social security number • Patient's full name and social security number • Membership, policy, certificate, or payroll numbers • Group number (if applicable), employer's name, address, and telephone number • Signed authorization for release of medical information at time of or after discharge • Policyholder's signature on assignment of benefits. • Effective date of policy • Pre-existing condition clause • Pre-certification number, if applicable • Other special requirements, if applicable • Dependent coverage • Signature on appropriate claimant's statement, if applicable
Commercial Individual	• Is assignment of benefits accepted? • Copy of card or policy • Dependent coverage • Pre-existing condition clause • Effective date • Pre-certification, if applicable • Other special requirements, if applicable • Policyholder's social security number and full name • Patient's social security number and full name • Claimant's statement signed and completed, if applicable • Required special forms signed and completed, if applicable

Helpful Hints—*Continued*

Coverage Type	Establish Verification and Check
Health Maintenance Organization/HMO	• If the hospital is not a regular provider, will the HMO pay the claim? • Copy of insurance I.D. • Is there a referral from an approved HMO physician? • Pre-certification, as applicable
Federal Group and Worker's Compensation	• See Blue Cross • See Commercial Group • See Worker's Compensation
Union Plans	• See Commercial Group • If union plan is self-insured, verify that assignment is accepted • Employment hours required for coverage (*important*) • Payroll number • Correct union information (name headquarters, identification number, etc.) is obtained
State Plan	• Sponsoring departmental voucher presented • Written or verbal approval from sponsoring agency (for verbal approvals, obtain patient identification number) • Hospital approved to render treatment for state sponsored patients
Charitable Organization	• Hospital approved to render treatment to charity sponsored patients • Organization will pay the hospital directly and honor an assignment of benefits. • Written approval is provided by the organization for the hospital to treat sponsored patient

Helpful Hints—*Continued*

Coverage Type	Establish Verification and Check
No Insurance (Self-Pay)	• Deposit collected or financed • Assignment of benefits is signed in case insurance becomes available • Business Office Manager or Inhouse Collector is notified immediately • Credit Bureau report is requested

On all insurance communication, always document comprehensively, clearly, and concisely.

III

Policies and Procedures

6

Policies and Procedures in Relation to Operations and Accounts Receivable

POLICY STATEMENT

Purpose

To establish responsibility for developing and implementing Accounts Receivable (A/R) controls.

Definition

Accounts Receivable—includes, but is not limited to, all facets of patient accounting procedure and asset management: pre-registration, pre-certification, registration, billing, collections, bad debts, utilization review, cost data collection and submission to required state agencies, etc., contract management, patient account inventory, A/R analysis, reporting, projections and information systems.

Responsibility

The Chief Financial Officer is responsible for all aspects of accounts receivable management, including development and documentation of hospital procedures specific to the community and facility operations. The A/R Manual represents *minimum* acceptable standards for A/R Management.

ADMISSION POLICY

Purpose

To ensure appropriate deposits are accurately determined and consistently collected at the time of admission or registration.

Policy

A deposit is necessary for patients with less than 100 percent verified insurance coverage. The amount of the expected deposit is calculated through use of the variable deposit method. Payment of the deposit can be made with cash, credit card, or check.

Exceptions to this policy should be approved in writing by hospital administration and made available to admitting personnel.

Calculation of Deposit

General Guidelines

Calculation of the deposit is based upon the variable deposit method. The amount required depends on the admitting diagnosis and anticipated surgical procedures, average hospital charges for that diagnosis, and the amount of verified third party coverage. (See *Variable Deposit Policy,* detailing methods for determining expected costs.)

If no information is available for that diagnosis, the hospital overall length of stay and average revenue per patient day are utilized to calculate the deposit.

Inpatient Deposit Requirements

Flat Rates—When a flat rate is agreed on (such as maternity, certain surgical procedures, etc.), payment is expected prior to but no later than the time of admission. Pre-admission deposits are encouraged and can be effectively managed as installment payments.

In cases where the patient has paid for a routine delivery and it is determined that a C-section is necessary, the patient will be billed for the difference. If agreed on payments are not made per policy, full charges are applicable and all previously quoted discounts nullified. Boarder baby charges will be billable.

Medicare Inpatient—No deposit is required for patients with verified secondary coverage. If no secondary coverage is available and annual deductible has not been met, the deductible is expected prior to discharge. Private room difference, if patient requested, is collected based on estimated length of stay.

Medicare Outpatient—No deposit is required for verified secondary coverage. If no secondary coverage is available, the deductible, if due, and 20 percent of charges (up to the annual maximum amount of patient responsibility), excluding all lab charges, are expected.

Medicaid—No deposit is required when coverage has been verified or other acceptable proof of eligibility is presented for the month of service. Applicable patient co-payments or share of cost is calculated and collected, when applicable.

Worker's Compensation—No deposit is required for verified worker's compensation admissions. The employer must be contacted for authorization and case number (if available). The authorizing party's name, insurance carrier, and billing address are documented. It is recommended that written verification be obtained in addition to telephone verification.

HMO—If the hospital is a contracted provider and has a referral from an approved HMO physician, no deposit is expected except for any co-insurance or deductible required under the coverage. If the hospital is not an authorized provider, the patient is considered self-pay.

PPO—A deposit is required for coinsurance and deductible. The amount is based on whether or not the hospital is an authorized PPO provider.

Champus—A deposit for coinsurance and deductible is expected. The amount is determined by the type of coverage—active or retired. If the patient does not have a non-availability form and the hospital is within 40 miles of a military medical facility, consider the patient self-pay.

Emergent/Urgent Admission—Patients deemed by the physician as emergent/urgent admits are advised of their financial responsibility and a deposit is requested based on the variable deposit criteria above. For emergent/urgent admissions, the deposit is not required prior to admission. Appropriate commitments are obtained regarding in-house payments, and so forth.

Non-Emergent/Urgent Verified Insurance—Patients admitted with coverage of less than 100 percent pay the balance equal to the portion of estimated total charges not covered by insurance.

Inpatients with coverage payable at 100 percent are not requested to pay a deposit.

Non-Emergent/Urgent Unverified Insurance—Admissions of non-emergent/urgent patients with unverified insurance should be delayed with the concurrence of the physician. Any patient admitted with unverified insurance is required to produce evidence of employment (I.D. badge, payroll check stub, insurance card) providing an indication of coverage. Patients with unverified coverage submit a *hold* deposit equal to the average total charges for that diagnosis. The patient is informed that the deposit will be held until insurance is verified with the appropriate amount returned or refunded, based on the benefits eventually verified.

If benefits are listed in the master insurance file, a deposit for deductible and co-insurance is expected based on information in the insurance master file, pending verification.

Non-Emergent/Urgent, Self-Pay—Patients without third party insurance coverage are required to pay applicable charges in full, or make payment arrangements if authorized.

Responsibility

It is the responsibility of the hospital Chief Financial Officer to implement and ensure adherence to the above admission policy. If it is deemed appropriate to waive the deposit requirements at admission, such exceptions should be made only by hospital administration or designee, and documented.

Insurance Verification Instructions

This information must be gathered for the verification process:

Verifier's Name: Employee performing the verification procedure.
Account Number: Unique computer number assigned to the patient.

Today's Date: Current month, day, year (MM/DD/YY).
Patient Name: Person receiving medical treatment.
DOB: Patient's date of birth (MM/DD/YY).
DX: Diagnosis provided by physician.
Procedure: Surgical procedure provided by physician.
Prim. Carrier: Insurance company to be initially responsible for payment of services rendered.
Insured: Policyholder's name (primary carrier).
Relationship: Policyholder's connection with patient, i.e., mother, brother, friend, and so forth.
SS#: Social Security number for person insured by primary carrier.
Pol#: Insurance identification number for person insured by primary carrier.
Grp#: Insurance group number for person insured by primary carrier.
Sec. Carrier: Secondary insurance responsible for payment on balance remaining once primary carrier has made payment.
Insured: Policyholder's name (secondary carrier).
Relationship: Secondary carrier policyholder's connection with patient (mother, brother, friend).
SS#: Social Security number for person insured by secondary carrier.
Pol#: Insurance identification number for person insured by secondary carrier.
Grp#: Insurance group number for person insured by secondary carrier.
Date of Accident: Date patient was injured (MM/DD/YY).
Location: Where the injury occurred (home, work, school, grocery store, etc.).

The basic benefits section must be verified with the insurance company and all items completed, when applicable. It is not necessary to ask if coverage is provided for well-baby coverage unless the mother is receiving treatment for pregnancy.

The primary insurance benefits are listed in the "Primary" column and secondary benefits in the "Secondary" column.

Complete as follows:

Basic Benefits

Effective Date: The date the insurance policy began (MM/DD/YY).
Pre-existing Wait Period: Some policies will not provide benefits for certain diagnoses for a predetermined period of time. Example: 12-month waiting period for maternity. This indicates there would be no benefits until the policy was in effect for a period of 12 months.
Exclusions: List any specific non-covered items stated by the insurance company.
Room and Board: Indicate the dollar amount or percentage the insurance company will pay daily for room and board services.
Ancillary: Indicate the dollar amount or percentage the insurance company will pay for ancillaries: lab, x-ray, pharmacy, and so forth.
Number of Days: The number of days for which coverage is provided.
Deductible: A defined dollar amount payable by the policyholder and deducted from the total charge prior to insurance payment.
Out-of-Pocket Expense: A defined dollar amount payable by the policyholder, usually required after a specified percentage has been paid and before further benefits are available.
Calendar Year Maximum: If applicable, the dollar amount and/or number of days limited by the insurance policy as a total payable benefit.
Lifetime Maximum: Dollar amount and/or number of days allowed by the policy. An example is diagnosed chemical dependency: insurance states the patient may receive treatment twice per lifetime, then no further benefits are available for that diagnosis.
Remaining Benefits: Dollar amount and/or number of days available if benefits have been previously paid for prior services.
Medical Records Required: Based on diagnosis, some insurance companies require a copy of the discharge summary, operative report, emergency room record, etc., to accompany the hospital's bill for services.
Coordination of Benefits: When the patient is covered by two insurance policies, it must be determined if the secondary policy will coordinate benefits with the primary policy in lieu of making duplicate payment, which would create a credit on the patient account.
Claim Form Needed: A special form unique to the insurance company, usually supplied to the patient by the insurance company or employer, must be completed by the patient in order to file it along with the UB-82 and itemized statement.
Second Opinion: A second physician or surgeon's opinion as related to the patient's condition.
Premiums Paid: Insurance premiums paid to a current status.
Verified With: (Name) The name of the person giving benefits from the insurance company.
Phone number of above: Telephone number of above person named.
Date verified: Actual date the insurance company was contacted for benefit information.
Well-baby coverage: Benefits for a healthy newborn with no complications.

Utilization Review

Review Organization: Name of the auditing party through which authorization for treatment of the patient must be obtained.

Phone number: Telephone number of person named above.

Authorization Number: Number obtained from the Review Organization, which must accompany the billing to the insurance company to verify proper authorization was obtained for services rendered.

Number of days authorized: Specified number of days authorized by the auditing party.

Date Authorized: Date (MM/DD/YY) authorization was obtained.

Authorized By: (Name) Name of person representing the Review Organization.

Concurrent Review: Some insurance companies require that they have availability to the patient's records, depending on diagnosis, during the course of treatment.

Billing Address: The address to which the hospital bill should be mailed.

Physician Benefits

Inpatient: Benefits that are applicable to payment of the doctor's bill for inpatient services.

Outpatient: Benefits that are applicable to payment of the doctor's bill for outpatient services.

Deposit Calculation

Estimated Length of Stay: Number of inpatient days expected for the diagnosis. This number is multiplied by the average daily revenue (hospital defined).

Estimated Surgery Cost: The total dollars estimated for a specific surgery.

Patient deductible, non-covered items, and co-insurance are payable by the patient. The amount should be indicated on the last line *Advance Payment Required.*

Variable Deposit Policy

Purpose

To ensure that deposits are accurately and consistently determined.

Policy

Deposits are collected at the time of registration for the self-pay portion after insurance has been verified. Administrative approval should be obtained if the balance is not collected at registration.

Procedure

The amount of deposit required depends on the admitting diagnosis, expected surgical procedures, and the amount of verified third party coverage. An accurate assessment of the patient's estimated length of stay and anticipated charges are essential to the deposit calculation.

There are various means of determining the estimated length of stay and anticipated charges. The most common methods are

- *Case-Mix System*—The hospital's automated medical records or grouper system can be used to supply diagnosis information versus average total charges.
- *In-Hospital Sampling*—Generally, the Medical Records Director is able to provide the Business Officer Manager a listing of the 25–35 most commonly used diagnoses and the average length of stay associated with each. This is the best method for determining average length of stay. The common diagnoses and average length of stay should be checked and updated regularly.

  The average charges for each of these diagnoses can be obtained by actual sampling of statements. With this information, the Registrars can be furnished with an alphabetized listing of the most commonly used diagnoses in the hospital, the corresponding average length of stay, and the anticipated charges by diagnosis and surgical procedure.
- *PAS Statistics Booklets*—PAS Statistics Booklets may be ordered from the Commission on Professional and Hospital Activities, Ann Arbor, Michigan (the Medical Records Department may have a copy of this booklet). These books provide information on lengths of stay by diagnosis for each geographical area; however, because the diagnoses are not listed in alphabetical order, information is difficult to access.
- *Physician's Estimates*—This method simply requires asking for the physician's estimation of the length of stay at the time of pre-registration or registration, which may be used in conjunction with inhouse sampling.

Insurance Verification

Verifier's Name ______________

Account # ______________ Today's Date: ______________

Patient Name: ______________ DOB: ______________

DX: ______________ Procedure: ______________

Prim. Carrier: ______________ Insured: ______________

Relationship: ________ SS # ________ Pol # ________ Grp # ________

Sec. Carrier: ______________ Insured: ______________

Relationship: ________ SS # ________ Pol # ________ Grp # ________

Date of Accident: ______________ Location: ______________

BASIC BENEFITS	PRIMARY		SECONDARY	
1. Effective Date:				
2. Pre-existing Wait Period:				
3. Exclusions:	Y/N		Y/N	Excl: ________
4. Room and Board:				
5. Ancillary:				
6. Number of Days:				
7. Deductible:				
8. Out-of-Pocket Expense:				
9. Calendar Year Maximum:	$ /	Dys	$ /	Dys
10. Lifetime Maximum:	$ /	Dys	$ /	Dys
11. Remaining Benefits:	$ /	Dys	$ /	Dys
12. Medical Records Required:	Y/N		Y/N	
13. Coordination of Benefits:	Y/N		Y/N	
14. Claim Form Needed:	Y/N		Y/N	
15. Second Opinion:	Y/N		Y/N	
16. Premiums Paid:	Y/N		Y/N	
17. Verified with: (Name)				
18. Phone Number of Above:				
19. Date Verified:				
20. Well-baby Coverage:	Y/N		Y/N	

UTILIZATION REVIEW	PRIMARY	SECONDARY
1. Review Organization:		
2. Phone Number:		
3. Authorization Number:		
4. Number of Days Authorized:		
5. Date Authorized:		
6. Authorized By: (Name)		
7. Concurrent Review:	Y/N	Y/N
8. Billing Address:		
To the Attention of:		

PHYSICIAN BENEFITS	PRIMARY	SECONDARY
1. Inpatient:		
2. Outpatient:		

DEPOSIT CALCULATION

Estimated Length of Stay ______________ × $ ________ = $ ________
Estimated Surgery Cost (if applicable): $ ________

Patient Deductible: (+) $ ______________
Non-covered items: (+) $ ______________
Co-insurance: (+) $ ______________

Advance Payment Required: $ ________

Once all the information has been gathered, all other important aspects are considered when establishing a variable deposit policy. The hospital's average charges per day must be determined so the deposit will be enough to cover the total amount of the bill.

When the patient's length of stay and the average daily charges for service have been estimated, any delinquent accounts with the hospital should be investigated. A delinquent account is any amount due the hospital from the patient or patient's family for past services for which agreed on arrangements are not in place. Delinquent accounts can be current or bad debt.

Any miscellaneous charges, such as private room difference and deductible due, should also be collected at the time of registration.

The total estimated charges for the services to be rendered are determined.

The average daily charge for the services rendered is multiplied by the estimated length of stay. (The average daily charges can be obtained from actual statement samplings.)

Step 1:	Average Daily Charge	×	Estimated Length of Stay	=	Total Estimated Charges

The amount covered by insurance or other third parties is subtracted from the total estimated charges determined in Step 1.

Step 2:	Total Estimated Charges	−	Verified Third Party Coverage	=	The Amount of Deposit Expected from Patient

If active account records and/or bad debt listings indicate that delinquent charges exist for that patient, any money owed from prior services is collected or satisfactory arrangements are made *before* future registrations are permitted. Miscellaneous charges such as patient-requested private room and personal or convenience items should also be collected. The amount for private room difference can be determined by multiplying the difference between a private room and a semiprivate room by the estimated length of stay. The amount of delinquent charges and the miscellaneous charges are added in Step 3. The sum will equal the expected deposit.

Step 3:	Total Estimated Charges	−	Verified Third Party Coverage	+	Amount of Delinquent Charges	+	Miscellaneous Charges	=	The Expected Deposit

Examples

A patient registers for a cholecystectomy, which has an average length of stay of two days. The average daily charges equal $800. Verification of the patient's third party coverage indicates that 80% of the charges will be covered, and no deductible is due. The patient has no past due accounts or any miscellaneous charges. The appropriate deposit for this patient is as follows:

Step 1:

Average Daily Charge		$ 800
× Estimated Length of Stay	×	2 days
= Total Est. Charges		$1,600

Step 2:

Total Est. Charges		$1,600
− Verified Third Party Coverage	−	1,280
		(80% of $1,600)
+ Delinquent Accounts	+	0
+ Miscellaneous Charges	+	0
= Total Required Deposit		$ 320

A prospective patient registers with an admitting diagnosis of diverticulitis, which has an estimated length of stay of five days. The average daily charges equal $800. Verification of the patient's third party coverage indicates 80% coverage with an unmet deductible of $100. The patient has a delinquent account of $120. The patient requests a private room; the private room difference is $20 per day.

Step 1:

Average Daily Charge		$ 800
× Estimated Length of Stay	×	5 days
= Total Est. Charges		$4,000

Step 2:

Total Est. Charges		$4,000
− Verified Third Party Coverage	−	3,120
		($4,000 − $100) × 80%
+ Delinquent Accounts	+	120
+ Miscellaneous Charges	+	200
= Total Required Deposit		$1,200

Deposit Computation

Patient Name ______________________________

Account # ______________________________

Admitting Clerk ____________ Date ____________

Step 1:

Average Daily Charge	$	________
× Estimated Length of Stay	×	________
= Total Estimated Charges (Or use hospital average charges for that particular diagnosis)	$	________

Step 2:

Total Estimated Charges	$	________
− Verified Third Party Coverage	−	________
+ Delinquent Account(s)	+	________
+ Miscellaneous (private room, deductible, etc.)	+	________
= Total Deposit Required	$	________

Registration Checklist

Purpose

To ensure that all aspects of the registration process (i.e., demographic and financial information obtained, copies of required documents made, signatures obtained, appropriate personnel notified, and forms distributed) are completed for every registration or admission.

Policy

The registration checklist is completed for each and every patient and should be completed in its entirety.

Procedure

- The Registrar completes a checklist for every registration.
- The checklist is filled out in its entirety. If an item does not apply to a patient, it is marked "N/A" for not applicable.
- If a required item or information could not be obtained, the Registrar explains the omission in the "comments" section of the checklist.
- Any additional pertinent information regarding the patient is explained in the "Comments" section.
- The checklist is filed in the patient's folder with all other paperwork.
- The Admitting Manager reviews the checklist for accuracy and completion while reviewing registrations.

Registration Checklist Definitions

The form is designed to enable the Registrar to simply check off most of the items, unless an explanation is required; it serves as a reminder to ensure all items are received from the patient.

Items on Checklist

- ID plate: patient charge plate.
- ID bracelet: patient identification bracelet.
- Log book: was the patient entered on the admit log?
- B.I.B.: brought in by (name of ambulance company).
- Patient info: information given to the switchboard or department responsible for patient information.
- ONG: overnight guest.
- Pre-admit? Indicate if the patient was pre-admitted.
- 23½: is the patient a 23½-hour observation patient?
- O/P doctor's orders: did doctor's orders accompany patient for diagnostic testing prescribed?
- W/C verified: is this a verified worker's compensation case?

Copies Made

- Insurance ID card(s): copy both sides of insurance identification cards because information such as mailing address for claims submission or benefits description is often printed on the back of the card.
- Driver's license: this is used to confirm correct address as well as provide picture identification of the patient.
- W/C auth: if worker's compensation, was authorization obtained and if so, is a copy of the authorization available?
- Dr's 1st rept: has the doctor's first report of injury been filed (in states where it is required)? Is a copy available for the patient file?

Medicare

- Medicare card: was a copy made?
- Part A: does the patient have hospital benefits?
- Effect date: effective date of Part A benefits.
- Part B: does the patient have medical insurance benefits?
- Effect date: effective date of Part B benefits.

- No card: there was no card available.
- U.R. notified: utilization review must be notified of all Medicare admissions.
- Medicare letter to pt: "Your Rights as a Medicare Patient" letter.
- MSP form: was Medicare Secondary Payor form completed?

Insurance

- Benefits verified: have benefits been verified with the insurance company or employer?
- Release: has the patient signed for release of information to insurance company?

Face Sheet

- Carrier codes: are the proper codes keyed for the insurance carriers?
- Financial class code: are the correct revenue codes keyed?
- Medical services: are the correct medical services codes keyed?
- Guarantor name and address: was this information obtained?
- Employer data: was this information obtained?

Deposits

- Collected: if collected, enter dollar amount here.
- Unable/refused (document): if the patient is unable to pay the requested deposit, give the reason why. Director of Admissions should be notified.
- Bad debt file checked: check the bad debt listing to see if the patient or any member of patient's family has previous bad debts that should be cleared prior to further treatment, unless an emergency.
- Open accts checked: check open accounts to see if the patient or any member of the patient's family has delinquent open accounts that should be cleared prior to further treatment, unless an emergency.

Signatures on Assignment

The patient signature must be obtained on assignments for the hospital, physician, pathologist, radiologist, and anesthesiologist in order to bill insurance for services rendered.

Insurance Copy

Distribute a copy of the insurance information to the folder, physician, pathologist, radiologist, and anesthesiologist for billing purposes.

Distribution

Forward a copy of the facesheet to

- Medical Records—Medical Records requires a copy of the facesheet for a permanent record of the patient's visits.
- X-Ray—for purposes of billing professional fees.
- Folder—for business office permanent record.
- M.D., Pathology, and Anesthesiology—for billing purposes.

Registered By

Name of the admitting clerk who registered the patient.

Distributed By

Name of admitting clerk who separated the paperwork.

Pre-Registration

Purpose

To obtain complete and accurate demographic and financial information and resolve any identified problems prior to the patient presenting for services to expedite the registration process.

Policy

Pre-registration is to be performed whenever the hospital has been notified at least 24 hours in advance of a pending registration or admission.

Procedure

The admitting physician (or physician's office) will call either the hospital surgical area or Admitting/Registration Office (preferred method of notification) to provide demographic, financial, and clinical information including:

- Patient name, address, telephone number, and social security number
- Patient birth date, age and gender
- Insurance information, including pre-certification or other special requirements such as second surgical opinion, and so forth.
- Employment information
- Physician name and telephone number
- Expected registration date

Registration Checklist

Patient Name: ______________________________ Date: ______________

ID Plate ____ ID Bracelet ____ Log Book ____ B.I.B. ______________________________

Patient Info _____ Pre-admit? y/n If not, could patient have been? ______ ONG ______________

23½ _____ O/P Doctor's Orders _____ W/C Verified _____

Copy of: Insurance ID Card(s) (both sides) __________ Driver's license ______________

W/C auth. __________ Dr's 1st Rept __________

M/Care: Medicare Card ______ Part A ______ Effect Date __________ Part B ______________

Effect Date ____________ No Card _________ U.R. Notified ______________

Medicare Letter to pt. __________ MSP Form __________

Insurance: Benefits Verified ______ Release ______

Facesheet: Carrier Codes _____ Fin. Class _____ Med. Serv. _____ Guarantor Name & Address _____ Employer Data _____

Deposits: Collected _____ Unable/refused _____

(document)____________________

Bad Debt File Checked _____ Open Accts Checked _____

Signatures on Assignment: Hospital __________ Physician __________ Path ______________

Rad _________ Anesth _________

Ins. Copy: Folder ______ Physician ______ Path ______ Rad ______ Anesth ______________

Distribution: (facesheet) Med Rec ________ X-ray ________ Folder ________ M.D. ______________

Path ________ Anesth ________

Registered by: ________________________ Distributed by: ______________________________

Comments:

- Admitting diagnosis and expected procedures (i.e., specific invasive operative procedures-operating room, or non-invasive operative procedures-treatment room)
- Pre-test (laboratory or radiology test), which must be performed as ordered by the physician

The Registrar ascertains whether the admitting physician is eligible to admit patients by checking the medical records suspension lists (see policy *Admitting Patients of Suspended Physicians*).

The information provided by the physician's office is keyed to the pre-registration screen and a copy printed to begin the patient account file. In facilities that do not have on-line admissions, the appropriate pre-registration form is manually completed.

Notify the UR Coordinator, or other appropriate personnel, immediately of all Medicaid admits and the proper authorization received.

Also, notify the UR Coordinator of all Medicare beneficiaries requiring PRO approval before *room assignment*.

Contact the patient immediately on receipt of the reservation.

All demographic and financial information is confirmed or added to the reservation form during contact with the patient.

Documentation included in the patient account file for all contact with prospective patients is to include no less than the following:

- Date
- Time
- Substance of contact
- Registrar's initials who performed the contact

Employment and insurance benefits are verified with the employer and/or insurance company once the pre-registration form is complete.

- Pre-certification, if required, is obtained if the physician has not already done so.
- Special requirements or approvals such as second surgical opinions are identified.
- Insurance coverage is clearly defined and documented for the type of service provided.
- Exceptions or limitations of insurance coverage are documented on the verification form so that the deposit requirement can be clearly defined for the patient upon arrival. This information is relayed to the patient during the second telephone call of the pre-admission process.

The registration deposit is calculated and documented prior to the second call to the patient. The variable deposit method is used to determine registration deposits.

The registration form is to be fully completed once all the demographic and financial information has been gathered and verified.

The pre-registered patient account file contains the following information:

- Pre-registration form
- Patient contact documentation
- Insurance benefits and eligibility
- Registration form completed, awaiting patient signatures upon arrival

The completed pre-registration patient account file is placed in the holding file under the expected registration date. (The holding file should consist of dividers numbered 1–31, representing the days of the month.)

A pre-admission log is maintained, indicating each patient's name, date expected, patient account number, and whether or not the insurance verification was performed. The Director of Admissions should check the log daily to ensure all pre-admits scheduled to be treated have had all necessary paperwork completed prior to the scheduled date of admission.

Psychiatric or other special treatment programs within the hospital are handled in this manner:

- When the program receives telephone calls or direct inquiries from prospective patients or referrals from private physicians, appointments for assessment sessions are scheduled. Assessments, for the purpose of this policy and procedure, are the same as pre-registration, and the same information is required, excluding any unrelated medical terminology (operative procedures, pre-tests).
- A pre-registration form is used to gather information during assessment if registration is done by the program personnel. The pre-registration form is forwarded to registration personnel for completion of the pre-registration process, which is the same as for acute patients.

Inpatient Admissions

Purpose

To obtain complete and accurate information while maintaining a very high public relations profile.

Policy

All components of the registration process are to be completed when the patient presents for admission.

Procedure

When a direct admit or pre-admitted patient presents at the admitting office, the Registrar ascertains whether the admitting physician is eligible to admit patients by checking medical records suspension lists (see policy on "Admitting Patients of Suspended Physicians").

The Registrar contacts the UR Coordinator or other appropriate personnel for all Medicare patients requiring PRO approval of the procedure (if not done during pre-admission) before room assignment.

The Registrar also immediately notifies the UR Coordinator or other appropriate personnel of all Medicaid admits and the proper authorization completed, when required (if not done during pre-admission).

Obtain all demographic and financial information, if not previously received.

Obtain all necessary signatures, to minimally include consent for admission and authorization to release information, and financial responsibility. If the insurance carrier requires a specific claim form, a signed copy must be obtained and placed in the patient's file. The hospital should stock claim forms for major payor and employer groups.

Make copies of the patient's driver's license, other I.D. and insurance cards, Medicare cards, Medicaid cards, and so forth, and place in the file.

Verify employer and insurance benefits with the employer and insurance company, if not previously done, while the patient is in the admitting office. Explain to the patient why verification is being done at that time.

- Pre-certification, if required, is to be obtained if the physician has not already done so.
- Special requirements or approvals such as second surgical opinions are identified.
- Insurance coverage needs to be clearly defined and documented for the type of service provided.
- Exceptions or limitations of insurance coverage are documented on the verification form so that deposit requirement can be clearly defined for the patient.

If the patient is Medicare, a Medicare Secondary Payor form must be completed to determine if Medicare is the primary payor, and the form filed in the patient financial file.

Calculate and request the deposit using the variable deposit method. If the patient cannot pay the deposit in full, refer the patient to the financial counselors, Director of Admissions or Business Office Manager, as appropriate, to make satisfactory arrangements.

- The Business Office Manager should have approval authority only on self-pay balances up to $1,000. If the balance exceeds $1,000, the account is to be referred to the Chief Financial Officer for his or her review to make the determination as to how the admission will be handled. Any account that has an estimated self-pay portion in excess of $3,000 should be referred to the Administrator for review and decision.
- Through each level of authority, there is documentation from the previous level. This ensures that all parties involved with receivables management are made aware of the type of account accepted.

If the patient is unable to pay the deposit or make satisfactory arrangements, the Business Officer Manager or Administrator notifies the physician of the patient's financial situation and asks if the admission can be rescheduled. If it can be delayed, the Business Office Manager notifies the patient. If the physician states that the patient needs immediate treatment, the patient is admitted without delay. All conversations with the patient and physician are to be fully documented on the financial file or in the system, as appropriate.

If the patient is Medicare, he or she must be given the form *Your Rights as a Medicare Patient.*

Obtain valuables, if applicable.

Assign the patient to a room, if Admitting is responsible for room assignment. Otherwise, notify nursing of the admission and obtain room assignment.

Place identification bracelet on the patient.

Notify the information desk and switchboard or other appropriate departments of the admission and room assignment as soon as possible.

Call Nursing for escort to the room.

Ensure that the correct revenue source code and all other codes are documented and keypunched properly.

Make and distribute all necessary copies of the face-sheet.

Place the financial folder in the appropriate location.

Complete the admission log.

Admitting Patients of Suspended Physicians

Purpose

To comply with hospital and medical staff policies regarding loss of clinical privileges of suspended physicians.

Policy

All direct and scheduled admissions should be ordered by physicians with current clinical privileges. It is the responsibility of the Registrar to review every direct and scheduled admission against the suspension list to ensure that the physician has current privileges. If an admission is ordered by a suspended physician, administrative approval must be obtained before the admission can be completed.

Procedure

The Medical Records department routinely provides suspension lists to the Director of Admissions, and the admitting, outpatient and ER registration areas.

Registrars review all pre-registrations at the time the reservation is received and again on the day of admission, and notify the Director of Admissions of all elective and direct admissions by suspended physicians.

The Director of Admissions telephones the Administrator, or a designee in his absence, for authorization before the admission process is initiated.

The Administrator makes the decision regarding authorization to admit. If authorization is denied, the Administrator notifies the physician of the decision.

If authorization is obtained, the Registrar completes the admission process and documents in the folder (or in the computer system) the name and title of the administrative person authorizing the admission, the date and time the authorization was obtained, and any other pertinent information.

If the admission is denied, the Registrar informs the patient that the admission process cannot be completed and tells the patient to contact his or her physician. The Registrar documents in the folder (or in the computer system) the name and title of the administrative person denying the admission, the date and time of the denial, and any other pertinent information.

Prior approval is not required for emergency admissions.

- For weekday emergency admissions, the Registrar notifies the Director of Admissions, who in turn, notifies the Administrator. The Registrar documents in the folder (or on the computer system) the date and time of the notification and any other pertinent information.
- For after hours emergency admissions, the Registrar telephones the administrative person on-call to notify of the admission. The Registrar documents in the folder (or in the computer system) the name and title of the administrative person notified, date and time of the call, and any other pertinent information.

Outpatient and Emergency Registrations

Purpose

To obtain complete and accurate information while maintaining a very high public relations profile.

Policy

All components of the registration process are completed when the patient presents for services.

Procedure

When the patient presents for treatment, ascertain whether it is for routine outpatient or emergency treatment.

If it is an emergency, notify physician or nursing personnel of the registration per hospital procedure.

The emergency room Registrar should never attempt triage of patient unless the Registrar is qualified to do so.

Obtain all demographic and financial information if possible. Obtain treatment authorization from certification group for HMO, PPO, etc., as appropriate.

If the patient requires immediate treatment, a limited amount of information can be obtained before the patient enters the treatment room. Generally, this information will be:

- Patient's name and address
- Age and date of birth
- Gender
- Date and time of registration
- Patient's family physician
- Chief complaint

Obtain all necessary signatures, at a minimum to include consent for treatment, authorization to release information, and financial responsibility.

Make copies of driver's license, other I.D., insurance cards, Medicare cards, Medicaid cards, etc., and place in the file.

If the patient has Medicare coverage, the Medicare Secondary Payor form must be completed, and a copy filed in the patient financial folder.

Verify employer and insurance benefits while the patient is in the registration area, if possible. The Insurance Master Index can be used to facilitate the verification process.

Verified insurance is acceptable for outpatients. Patients with coverage of less than 100 percent are expected to pay the balance equal to the estimated portion not covered by insurance. The patient is also expected to pay the deductible, if due.

Outpatients with unverified insurance are required to make payment in full for services rendered and insurance is then billed as a courtesy, or services may be delayed until verification is possible.

The hospital may want to establish a minimum dollar amount for accepting insurance. Payment in full would be expected for charges less than the minimum amount (excluding Medicare, Medicaid, worker's compensation, Blue Cross, HMO, and Champus).

Full payment is expected for emergency room charges, based on the charge master. A flat rate deposit is paid at the time of registration, and final payment made after service is rendered.

If active account records or bad debt listings indicate that delinquent charges exist for the patient or patient's family, the Registrar should attempt to collect the unpaid balances.

Under no circumstances should a patient requesting emergency service be refused due to their inability to meet the financial requirements of the hospital.

The Registrar should notify patients they will be billed separately by the physicians, unless physician charges are included in the facility's charges.

Obtain valuables, if applicable.

Place an identification band on the patient, if applicable.

Direct patients to the treatment area. Emergency, stretcher, and wheelchair patients should be escorted by nursing personnel, volunteers, or other designated personnel.

Ensure that the correct revenue source code and all other codes are documented and keypunched properly.

Copy and distribute facesheets.

Place financial file in the appropriate location.

Complete the registration log.

When it is determined that an E.R. patient or outpatient will be admitted as an inpatient, follow the procedure below.

- Transfer the patient from E.R. or outpatient status to inpatient status and follow applicable procedures to transfer charges to an inpatient account.
- Notify Admitting of the admission.
- Print (if the facility has on-line admission) or type inpatient facesheet if different forms are used for inpatient admissions.

- The Registrar performs the insurance verification and admission authorization, if required. Facilities using a separate person to verify should implement controls to ensure verification is completed in time to make financial arrangements.
- Send the patient's folder to admitting.

Recurring Outpatients

Purpose

To obtain complete and accurate demographic and financial information on recurring outpatient; and to establish controls to ensure billing is performed consistently and the patient is discharged appropriately when treatment has been completed.

Policy

All aspects of the registration process are performed at the time of the initial visit for patients for whom a definite and repeated treatment program is established. No department renders service unless proof of registration is provided by the patient.

The account is billed monthly on an interim basis until the time of discharge.

Procedure

Registration

Recurring outpatients are registered at the time of the initial visit by the pre-admission clerk or registration clerk. All demographic and financial data is obtained as well as consent for treatment, deposits/deductibles collected, and prescriptions checked.

Manual systems utilize 3 × 5 cards with the patient name, number, and date of registration; the cards are filed alphabetically in a card file.

Patient type is listed as recurring and the patient folder marked accordingly. If a separate patient class is not used for recurring outpatients, another method should be used to differentiate these patients from regular outpatients.

Payment in full or acceptable insurance verification is to be obtained during the initial registration process.

The patient is sent to the appropriate department with physician orders and a copy of the facesheet or other form of notification indicating the account number. Services cannot be rendered if this does not accompany the patient.

When the patient arrives for subsequent visits, the 3 × 5 card file is checked. If a card exists for the patient, it indicates that the patient is a recurring account. The account number and patient name is written on a charge ticket or other form of notification, and given to the patient. If a 3 × 5 card does not exist, it indicates the patient is not a recurring account and will have to be registered as a new patient.

The financial folder is routed to the Director of Admissions for review the day following registration.

Worker's compensation accounts will be reverified every month until discharge.

If a patient, including a nursing home patient, maintains status as a recurring patient for ninety days, the account is manually discharged and re-registered by asking the patient for all demographic information to obtain any updated information.

Discharge

At discharge, the department sends a completed discharge slip to the cashier or discharge clerk, with a copy to Medical Records.

The cashier or discharge clerk keys in the discharge date for on-line systems, or sends the discharge slip to data processing if the facility does not have automated ADT. A final bill is printed. Order entry on-line systems can produce an immediate final bill.

Interim billing is done at the end of each month until discharge; the patient's account number, however, does not change.

The cashier or discharge clerk sends the discharge slip to the business office for filing in the financial folder.

Any account with no charge activity for 30 days is discharged, final billed, and the appropriate department is notified. The computer system should be profiled, if possible, to automatically discharge these patients; the procedure can, however, be performed manually.

When the final bill comes off the system, the corresponding 3 × 5 card for that bill is pulled and thrown away.

23-Hour Observation

Purpose

To provide an outpatient observation status for Medicare patients whereby they may be observed, before admission to the hospital, to determine whether the patient meets PRO criteria for an inpatient admission, requires observation following a procedure, or needs to be stabilized for safe discharge.

To avoid non-covered inpatient admissions and to maintain review status with the PRO and avoid Medicare sanctions for inappropriate hospital admissions.

Definition

23-Hour patients are

- Those with a medical need that may or may not require acute hospitalization. Testing and observation can be performed for patients with vague or questionable symptoms, enabling the physician to gather information to determine the degree of medical necessity for further hospitalization on an acute inpatient basis.
- Those patients with a medical need that can be safely and effectively evaluated or treated on an outpatient basis with short-term aggressive treatment and nursing observation.
- Patients who are social cases, not medically requiring acute care but in need of skilled nursing care, who must be hospitalized.

This classification provides the physician with more time to decide whether acute level of care is appropriate for a certain select number of patients who present with signs and symptoms that require treatment but who may not meet established Medicare guidelines for covered services in the acute hospital setting.

The 23-Hour Hold Program is an expansion of the hospital's outpatient service, to allow for evaluation, observation, and implementation of treatment of a select group of patients within the acute hospital setting for a defined period of time (less than 24 hours).

Policy

In response to the changes in Medicare regulations and to determinations by the PRO that certain admissions have been medically unnecessary (the patient could have been safely and effectively treated on an outpatient basis), the hospital has developed an outpatient classification called "23-Hour Hold Patient."

The hospital will provide beds on inpatient nursing units that may be utilized by staff physicians for *outpatient observation* of unstable Medicare patients who may later require admission. Bed assignment will be made on the same basis as a regular inpatient admission.

Outpatients may be held in this status or classification for up to 23 hours and 59 minutes before a final decision to admit or discharge is made. If the Medicare patient is admitted, the date and time of admission are when the patient originally entered the facility for treatment.

Procedure

The physician notifies Admitting that the Medicare patient is to be observed and specifies the type of room requested.

Admitting assigns an observation room or calls nursing for room assignment and notifies the Utilization Review Coordinator (URC). The "Outpatient Observation Letter" is given to the patient or family member.

In addition to an identifiable arm band and charge plate, observation patients are registered with a selected numeric sequence to further identify the patient type.

The URC notifies Admitting, after the observation period is up, as to whether the patient will be released or is to be admitted.

If the patient is to be admitted, the family is sent to the admitting office to admit the patient. If no family member is available, Admitting will do a bedside admit.

Medicare patients who are admitted will have their charges converted to an inpatient status, and costs will be reimbursed on the basis of the DRG. No charge is made for hourly observation because the daily room rate covers that service.

Discharged Medicare patients will be billed for charges incurred, including emergency visit, any services performed, and observation time. The hospital accepts a Medicare assignment for covered services and bills Part B. The patient is billed for any unmet deductibles and the co-insurance. Medically necessary observation time is chargeable on an hourly basis.

The patient file folders are reviewed daily by the Director of Admissions to ensure all procedures were correctly followed by all personnel concerned.

The medical record requirements of the physician are the same as those of an E.R. record if the patient is not admitted. If the patient is admitted, the medical record requirements of the physician are the same as those of an inpatient.

Records of patients who have been in *outpatient observation* and are subsequently discharged are filed with emergency or outpatient records. Records of patients who are admitted, having been in outpatient observation, are filed with inpatient records.

Outpatient Observation Letter

Dear Patient & Family Member:

You or one of your family members has been admitted to the Outpatient Observation Program of our hospital. The program is designed to serve our Medicare patients and is our way of assisting in controlling inpatient health care costs. Outpatient Observation is utilized when it cannot be determined after evaluation in the emergency department if an extended admission will be necessary. The patient will be placed on a regular nursing unit and monitored, but will remain an outpatient. A patient may remain in Outpatient Observation for up to 23 hours, following arrival. The patient may have testing done, receive medications, or just be monitored. At the conclusion of 23 hours, or sooner, the physician will determine if the patient should be admitted as an inpatient for further care or discharged from this status.

Family members do not have to remain with the patient, but they should be available to hospital personnel within an hour's notice so that the patient may be taken to his or her place of residence if dismissed. Medicare regulations require the patient be classified as an admission if he or she physically stays over 24 hours in a hospital. The patient will be required to pay the inpatient deductible, if applicable, if the stay exceeds 24 hours. *If an admission is necessary,* a family member should be available to complete admission paperwork, if the patient is not able to do so. If the patient is able to make decisions for himself or herself, has necessary information, and has no family member present, admitting personnel will perform a bedside admission.

When the patient is discharged from Outpatient Observation, charges incurred for any services will be filed with Medicare (Part B) or other insurance for outpatient services, if the patient has such outpatient benefits. The patient will be responsible for unmet deductibles and co-insurance following Medicare or other insurance consideration.

If an admission is necessary, all charges incurred in the emergency department and during observation will be covered by the reimbursement the hospital receives for inpatient care.

Thank you for choosing our hospital and we hope we can make your stay comfortable.

Administration

Medicare Pre-admission Review Requirements

Purpose

To ensure adherence to Medicare regulations for those procedures requiring pre-admission authorizations.

Policy

Medicare regulations state that pre-admission authorization is required for certain procedures that have been designated as "Elective/Scheduled," if Medicare is the primary payor. Prior to admission, required authorization must be obtained.

- Patients scheduled to be admitted from an acute PPS hospital to certain facilities, such as exempt psychiatric hospital or unit, exempt physical rehabilitation hospital or unit, alcohol or other chemical dependency rehab hospital or unit, or swing bed in an acute facility.
- Services involving level of care criteria.
- Services involving medical necessity criteria.

Procedures

Procedures involving level of care and medical necessity criteria can be scheduled on an outpatient basis without need of authorization. If any of these procedures are performed on an emergent basis in conjunction with other medical emergency problems, authorization is not necessary.

Only the physician can call and obtain authorization. The hospital cannot call on the physician's behalf.

The authorization must be obtained from PRO before admission because authorization requests received after the patient's admission to the hospital will not be processed.

The physician contacts PRO to obtain authorization.

The physician's office forwards documentation from PRO confirming the authorization to Admitting for inclusion in the patient's folder.

Admitting provides Utilization Review with a copy of the authorization.

If authorization has not been obtained by the time the patient presents for service, the physician will be notified and the admission delayed until authorization is received.

Medicare Re-admissions and Transfers

Purpose

To ensure adherence to Medicare requirements regarding the re-admission and transfer of Medicare patients.

Policy

Medicare regulations state that PRO be notified of re-admission and transfer of Medicare patients. The admitting hospital is responsible for completing the "Review Notification Form" and submitting it to the PRO office responsible for the review within one working day of the re-admission or transfer.

In the case of transfers, notify the PRO of any transfers from a PPS hospital to any other acute hospital or to an exempt hospital.

Procedure

Transfers

When pre-admitting a patient who is being transferred from another facility, the reason for transfer is noted to ensure that applicable pre-admission requirements are met.

After admission into the receiving hospital, the U.R. Coordinator or other designated personnel is notified and is responsible for completing the notification form and forwarding it to PRO.

Re-admissions

All Medicare admissions should be screened by Admitting to identify when the patient was last hospitalized. The dates of admission and discharge should be recorded in the financial file.

Re-admissions within the last 30 days must be identified, including patients discharged from any other acute care hospital in the United States.

After admission, the U.R. Coordinator or other designated personnel are notified and are responsible for completing the notification form and forwarding it on to PRO within one working day of the date the hospital becomes aware of the re-admission.

Copies of the notification form are filed in the patient's financial file and utilization review file.

Sterilization Consents for Medicaid Patients

Purpose

To ensure that state regulations regarding elective sterilization procedures on Medicaid patients are followed.

Policy

Sterilization consents for Medicaid patients must be signed by the patient at least 30 days prior to an elective sterilization procedure. The consents must be received by the admitting department before the patient is admitted or registered. No patient will be admitted without a signed sterilization consent on file.

Procedure

Sterilization consents are received from the admitting physician prior to the admission date.

After registration, a copy of the sterilization consent is maintained in the financial folder. The original is attached to the medical chart and accompanies the patient to surgery.

If there is no consent on file when the patient presents for admission, notify the physician that the admission cannot be completed until proper consent is received.

Personal Injury/Worker's Compensation Liens

Purpose

To ensure that the appropriate actions are taken to protect the hospital's interests.

Policy

It is at the hospital's discretion to accept patients covered under personal injury or worker's compensation liens. All liens must receive approval from administration.

A guarantee is required from the patient's attorney that the hospital's interests will be protected and a lien signed by both the attorney and patient, along with the hospital defined advance deposit. If these are not obtained, the account will be considered self-pay and full payment expected at registration or treatment will be delayed with concurrence of the physician and administration.

Procedure

The physician contacts Admitting to schedule treatment and provide the following information:

- Diagnosis
- Procedure
- Insurance information
- Attorney's name
- Date of injury
- Admission date

The Registrar contacts the patient and obtains:

- All demographic information
- Employment information
- Any group insurance
- Confirmation of information given by the physician

The Registrar contacts the patient's attorney and informs him or her of the hospital's policy regarding the acceptance of liens.

For worker's compensation cases, the state worker's compensation agency's notice of claim or lien form signed by the patient at the time of admission, then completed by the business office and forwarded for the attorney's signature prior to admission. Copies of the lien are distributed to the state worker's compensation appeals board, insurance carrier, attorney, employer, patient and hospital file.

In personal injury cases, a letter of guarantee should be completed and signed by the attorney and received by the hospital prior to admission.

Numeric Admit Type Code for UB-82/Medical Records Compliance

Purpose

To comply with state and federal regulations as well as UB-82 requirements.

Policy

An alpha admission type code should be identified on all admissions by using the following criteria:

CODE	DEFINITION (CONDITION OF PATIENT)
1	EMERGENCY: Patient requires immediate medical intervention as a result of severe, life threatening or potentially dis abling conditions. Generally, the patient is admitted through the emergency room.
2	URGENT: Patient requires immediate attention for the care and treatment of a physical or mental disorder. Generally the patient is admitted to the first available and suitable accommodation.
3	ELECTIVE: Patient's condition permits adequate time to schedule the availability of a suitable accommodation.

Canceled Admissions/Registrations

Purpose

To ensure that all canceled admissions and registrations are deleted at the time of notification.

Policy

Admitting is to be notified by the appropriate department on a timely basis of all patients who have been registered but do not receive treatment due to appointment cancellation or the patient not showing.

Admitting is responsible for monitoring the pre-admissions report to ensure that all cancellations or no-shows have been reported and appropriately deleted.

Procedure

The appropriate ancillary department or emergency room staff informs admitting via canceled charge ticket, order entry or some other form of notification.

The cancellation notification is placed in the patient folder, and the facesheet pulled from the daily work. The folder is placed with the regular patient folders for review by the Director of Admissions, then forwarded to the business office to be filed.

The Director of Admissions ensures that the pre-admissions report is reviewed weekly for past due pre-admissions. The appropriate ancillary department, pre-admission clerk, or physician's office is contacted to determine the status of the admission.

- If the patient canceled or did not show, the above procedures will be performed.
- If the date of service has been changed, the pre-admission file and/or computer system is updated to show the new expected date.

Discharge

Purpose

To ensure that all patients obtain financial clearance before leaving the hospital.

Policy

All patients discharged from the hospital obtain financial clearance and release from the cashier or discharge office, if a courtesy discharge has not been issued prior to discharge. It is the responsibility of the nursing staff to ensure that such a release is obtained. It is the responsibility of the cashier or discharge clerk to ensure that discharge interviews are handled professionally to create an efficient, courteous, and pleasant experience for the patient.

Procedure

Discharge Office or Cashier

The discharge clerk or cashier prints or receives a listing of in-house patients daily. This report lists admit date, patient balance to date, and patient length of stay.

Using the list of pending discharges obtained from the nursing units, the discharge clerk or cashier:

- Pulls the patient files from admitting.
- Reviews the patient insurance verification forms for benefits.
- Computes patient share of cost (if not done at admission) as follows:
  1. deductible, if any
  2. co-insurance, if any
  3. deduct any payments received, such as deposit
- Adds up the total estimated balance due from the patient or guarantor and notes the amount on the patient file folder.

When nursing staff escorts the patient to the discharge office or cashier's office, the discharge clerk or cashier:

- Pulls the patient financial file.
- Reviews the benefits.
- Collects any balance due from the patient, as computed above.
- Explains to the patient that any payment made at that time is based on only an estimate of the total charges.
- Directs the patient to financial counselors, Director of Admissions or Business Office Manager, if the patient is unable to pay the share of cost.

Nursing Staff

- Completes the discharge slip or enters the information into the system computer.
- Escorts the patient to the discharge clerk or cashier, if a courtesy discharge has not been issued, or sends the patient's guarantor as shown on the facesheet to the discharge clerk/cashier for financial clearance and release.
- Escorts the patient out of the hospital when the financial release is received from the discharge clerk or cashier.

Courtesy Discharge

Purpose

To promote positive public relations by providing an expeditious discharge process for those patients who meet all financial obligations prior to discharge.

Policy

When benefits have been verified at 100 percent coverage or another acceptable level, or the patient has paid the balance or made satisfactory arrangements, and all signatures have been obtained, a courtesy discharge letter is issued to the patient. The letter states that the patient does not need to stop by the discharge office or business office at the time of departure, unless there are patient valuables to collect. Nursing should ensure the patient receives the letter at time of discharge.

Procedure

Admitting provides nursing with the courtesy discharge letter.

Nursing files the letter in the patient's chart, and gives it to the patient at the time of discharge.

Courtesy Discharge Letter

Dear ______________________________:

I hope your stay at our hospital was as comfortable as possible.

You have met all of the financial requirements for discharge, therefore, you will not need to stop by our discharge office, unless you have valuables to collect, when you have been released by your physician.

Upon notification by nursing service, you may leave the hospital directly from your room with a courtesy discharge.

I would like to take this opportunity to express my sincere appreciation to you for selecting our hospital and its medical staff for your health care needs.

Sincerely,

Administration

Census Balancing

Purpose

To ensure that the census statistics are accurately reported daily.

Policy

The census will be balanced with the computer system and medical records accurately and timely on a daily basis.

Procedure

A pre-list is run daily, including all admissions, discharges, and transfers.

The pre-list is forwarded to Nursing for verification and actual head count, then returned to Admitting to confirm the accuracy of the manual or computerized bed board (if admitting is responsible for controlling the bed board).

When the accuracy of the pre-list is confirmed, the final census is printed and distributed to all appropriate departments.

If the census does not balance, the Director of Nursing is responsible for ensuring the error is corrected.

The Business Office manager notifies the Chief Financial Officer if there are continuing problems with census balancing.

Chart Flow from Admitting

Purpose

To outline the flow of discharged financial folders from the admitting area to the Business Office.

Policy

Discharged financial folders are to be accounted for by the registration areas and sent to the business office daily with copies of registration sheets attached.

Procedure

Discharged financial folders are received in the business office one day after discharge.

The folders are routed from Admitting with a copy of the registration log and discharge report attached.

Director of Admissions:

- Reviews the discharge report daily as a quality control measure to assure that inpatient financial folders indicating as discharges match the daily inpatient discharges. Any discharged financial folders being held in Admitting are indicated on the discharge report with the name of the admitting personnel holding the folder, and an outcard is submitted in lieu of the financial folder.
- Ensures that files are accounted for and ready for Business Office by 9:00 A.M. one day after discharge. All files are reviewed by the Director of Admissions to ensure all procedures were correctly followed. For after hours and weekend patients, folders are reviewed for the required deposits until insurance verification can be done.
- Routes the relative discharged financial folders and outcards to the Business Office Manager.
- Maintains and updates copies of the discharge report and ensures all folders are received in lieu of the outcards in a timely manner.

Business Office Manager

- On receipt of the discharged inpatient financial folders and outcards, reviews the folders and outcards for completeness and accuracy and ensures all folders are accounted for.
- After review, the files are kept in an inhouse tub awaiting final bills.

Matching Bills to Folders

Purpose

To ensure that every financial folder receives a bill and that a bill exists for each folder.

Policy

All bills are compared to the billing report and matched to folders before billing.

Procedure

Discharged accounts are filed alphabetically by date of discharge in the pending bills file.

When bills are produced, they are checked against the billing report to ensure all bills are accounted for. All discrepancies are given to the Business Office Manager for immediate resolution.

The bills are broken apart and matched to folders to ensure that a folder exists for each bill. All discrepancies are brought to the Business Office Manager for immediate resolution.

After all discrepancies are resolved, the files and bills are routed to the appropriate department for billing.

Late Charges

Purpose

To ensure that all late charges are appropriately billed or adjusted off accounts.

Policy

All late charges will be billed or adjusted off accounts when the late charge is received. All billings are reviewed by the Business Office Manager and compared to the late charge report to ensure that the appropriate action was taken. The Business Office Manager keeps a record of all late charges and presents it to the Chief Financial Officer on a weekly basis.

Procedure

A late charge report is received daily by the billers and a copy forwarded to the Business Office Manager.

The report is given to the file clerk to run inquiries on the accounts and pull the patient files.

The folders are placed in the appropriate area for rebilling.

Necessary adjustments are made.

- *Duplicate Charges:* The ancillary department is contacted to determine how the charges were duplicated and if they are legitimate. By checking daily batching against the department log for services rendered, this should not occur.
- *Flat Rates:* If the initial adjustment was made for an approved flat rate account, the late charges also should be adjusted to bring the account to a zero balance. Paid ER/OP accounts are adjusted the same way.

- *Medicare I/P Late Charges:* If the account has been billed to Medicare and then additional charges are submitted from the ancillary departments, the charges should be written off as Medicare late charges and logged in the Medicare Late Charge log.
- *HMO/PPO Late Charges:* If payment to the hospital is a per-diem payment, the late charges should be written off to the appropriate write-off code. If payment is a percentage payment, the late charges are billed to the insurance carrier.
- *All Other Late Charges:* Bill as additional charges to the proper insurance carrier on a copy of the original UB-82 so the carrier will know this is not duplicate billing.

The late charge report and patient files are forwarded to the Business Office Manager for review.

The Business Office Manager discusses late charges with the offending departments and notifies the Chief Financial Officer if the late charge problem is not corrected.

Secondary and Supplemental Insurance Billing

Purpose

To ensure all appropriate balances are billed to the secondary insurance on a timely basis.

Policy

All secondary insurances are to be billed when the remittance advice or notification of payment is received in the Business Office.

Procedure

All remittance advices are forwarded to the Billing Supervisor, or other designated personnel, from the cashier.

The remittance advices are given to the file clerk to make copies, run inquiries, and pull the files with remaining balances.

The files are forwarded to the Billing Supervisor, or designated staff person, for delegation to the billers. The Billing Supervisor ensures that all files with balances were actually pulled.

Unlocated files are indicated on the remittance advices and pulled the next day.

Over-the-Counter Collections

Purpose

To establish cash controls for payments made at the hospital.

Policy

Cash receipts are used to record payments and issue receipts over the counter. Carbon images of the receipt can be used as keypunch documents to process cash receipts. The original receipt is given to the payor.

Procedure

When the cashier is closed, other registration personnel may be designated to accept cash payments from patients. The responsibility includes:

- Maintaining custody of the cash box and cash drawer keys for the entire shift
- Issuing receipts for all payments with receipts in strict numeric order
- Maintaining a cash receipts journal
- Balancing all monies with incoming employee
- Depositing all monies into the drop safe at the end of shift
- Documenting and signing shift totals in cash log
- Notifying department manager and/or house supervisor of any discrepancies
- Maintaining these collections as accounts receivables only, not to be used for petty cash, making change, or cashing checks

The cash drawer is counted and reconciled at the beginning and end of each shift by both the cashiers and the Registrars coming on and ending their shifts.

Each transaction is documented in a cash receipts journal and submitted with cash collections on each shifts.

A written numbered receipt slip is issued for all payments received. Numbered receipts are kept in numeric order at all times.

Corrections are made by voiding the receipt slip and neatly marking one line through the information to be changed on the hospital's cash receipts journal.

Copies of all voided receipt tickets are stapled to the cash sheet.

Credit cards are treated as cash.

All checks are restrictively endorsed by stamping the back of check with the hospital's endorsement.

All currency and checks are kept in the locked cash drawer until the end of each shift.

A cash receipts journal is completed and balanced at the end of each shift, and the daily log is signed by both registrars and cashiers.

The cash receipts journal and monies collected are put into the drop safe at the end of each shift.

Any discrepancies are reported immediately to the department manager or House Supervisor, who will notify administration.

Daily Cashier Reconciliation and Recap

The Daily Cashier Reconciliation and Recap is a report completed by the hospital cashier on a daily basis to reconcile the cash drawer for the bank deposit and recap the over-the-counter and mail cash for the day.

The Daily Cashier Reconciliation and Recap is divided into sections as follows:

- *Amount in Drawer:* At the end of the work day as the cashier closes, the total amount of cash and checks collected are documented in the left column. The right column represents the amount of cash equaling the base amount for the next day.
- Reconcile—Cashier:

  Total Amount in Drawer: This figure is derived from section A where the total amount of cash and checks is totaled.

  OTC Checks: All OTC checks are separated and totaled here.

  Mail Checks: All mail checks are separated and totaled here.

  Total Cash on Hand: All mail and OTC cash is separated and totaled here and should equal the following formula:

  Total Amount in Drawer − OTC Checks − Mail Checks = Total Cash on Hand

- *Total Receipts:* All A/R patient cash receipt postings and miscellaneous cash receipt postings, sum totaled and the figure placed here.
- *Amount of Cash Drawer:* The total base amount of the drawer is placed here.
- *Balance:* For the Cashier to balance, the following formula should be used:

  Total Amount in Drawer − Total Receipts − Amount of Cash Drawer = 0.00

  The total must equal zero to make certain that all cash was properly posted.
- *Recap—Cashier:* Once the cash drawer has been properly reconciled in sections A and B, the cashier must recap the types of cash flow.

  Over-the-Counter: The cash posted as OTC should tie with the Collection Recap—OTC.

  Mail: The cash posted as mail should tie with the Business Office Cash Flow Recap and is derived from the total of the Cash Receipts Posting posted exclusively for mail cash.

  Misc. Cash Receipts: This figure represents total cash collected from sources usually non-patient, such as dietary services and vending machine commission.

  Total Deposit: The sum of the above receipts equals the total bank deposit for the day.

  Date: The cashier must date this report and attach copies of the bank deposit and cash receipt journals used in the reconciliation for future record-keeping.

  - *Reconcile—Admitting Clerk:* This recap is exclusively for use if an admitting clerk or second shift cashier re-opens the cash drawer prior to the next business day.

Cashier

DAILY CASH RECONCILIATION AND RECAP

Amount in Drawer		Recap—Cashier		
Pennies	________	Over the Counter	=	________
Nickels	________			
Dimes	________	Mail	=	________
Quarters	________			
½ Dols.	________	Misc. Cash Rec.	=	________
Dollars	________			
Fives	________	*Total Deposit	=	________
Tens	________			
Twenties	________	Date		________
________	________			
Cashed Checks	________	Cashier Name:		________
Total Amt. in Drawer	________			

________ - ________

Reconcile—Cashier			Reconcile—Admit Clerk		
Total Amt. in Drawer	$	________	Total Amt. in Drawer	$	________
OTC Checks	−	________	Total Receipts	−	________
Mail Checks	−	________	**Balance	=	________
Total Cash on Hand	=	________	(** should = Amount of Cash Drawer)		
*Total Receipts	−	________	Clerk Initials ________ Date ________		
Amt. of Cash Drawer	−	________	Incoming Clerk ________ Date ________		
**Balance	=	________			

(* Should = total daily recap)
(** Should = 0.00)

Cash Receipts/Collections

Week ending: ____________

Attach copy of Daily Cash Report for the last day of the week's reporting period. This report must tie with bank deposit/AR posting summary.

Number and Amount of Accounts Receivable:

Number: ______________________ Amount: $ ______________________

In-House Collector Activity:

NAME (Full-time)	# CALLS	AMOUNT OF BILLS	AVERAGE AMOUNT
1. ____________	________	____________	____________
2. ____________	________	____________	____________
3. ____________	________	____________	____________
4. ____________	________	____________	____________
TOTALS:	________	____________	____________
GOAL:	________		

COMMENTS: ____

____

____

____

TOTAL UP-FRONT DEPOSITS (e.g. Cash, Credit Cards):

$ ______________________

TOTAL CASH COLLECTED FROM IN-HOUSE PATIENTS:

$ ______________________

PROJECTED BAD DEBT (SELF-PAY) ADMISSIONS (Est. over $3,000)

PATIENT INITIALS	DIAGNOSIS	DEPOSIT PAID
____________	____________________	$ ____________________
____________	____________________	$ ____________________
____________	____________________	$ ____________________
____________	____________________	$ ____________________
____________	____________________	$ ____________________

Balancing Cash to Daily Deposit

Purpose

To establish strict cash controls for incoming cash.

Policy

All incoming cash is to be balanced and deposited on a daily basis.

Procedure

The daily deposit is made of all cash received since the last cash cutoff period.

All records of miscellaneous (non-patient) cash receipts are accumulated.

All amount received figures and all miscellaneous cash monies are totaled. This sum must balance to the total daily deposit figure.

After the financial manager verifies that cash is in balance, it is submitted to data processing for keying or entered in the on-line system.

After A/R update, the A/R general ledger posting is reviewed and the balances in all general ledger cash accounts sum to the daily deposit total are verified.

Any reconciliation necessary to achieve the balance is performed.

Cash posting documentation with handwritten notations confirming the balance is filed.

Returned Checks

Purpose

To establish guidelines for the proper processing of returned checks.

Policy

A log is to be maintained for returned checks. All checks returned for insufficient funds are logged in, redeposited the day after receipt, and follow-up procedures are initiated with the patient or guarantor.

Procedure

The returned check is logged in.

The check is redeposited and the patient advised of the situation.

If the check is returned twice, it is charged back to the patient account.

The appropriate bank is notified that a check is being sent to them for collection. The bank holds the check for a pre-determined amount of time and deposits it when funds are available in the account.

The returned check is photocopied and forwarded to the Business Office Manager for distribution to collectors.

Cash Posting

Purpose

To ensure accurate and timely processing and depositing of all cash receipts. To ensure payments are posted to the appropriate general ledger and patient account numbers, and contractual adjustments are applied at the time of receipt.

Policy

All cash and checks, whether identified or not, are to be balanced, deposited, and posted to the appropriate account daily. The cashier is responsible for processing all cash receipts, applying contractual adjustments, and processing physician payments.

(For the purpose of this policy, the term "checks" will also encompass check copies if a lock box system is utilized.)

Procedure

The hospital mail is collected daily and sorted by the cashier, who separates the checks from all other mail. The checks are processed by the accounts payable clerk or a designated employee other than the cashier. The checks are removed from each individual envelope and clipped to the same for ease of payor identification. A total of all checks is produced. Checks and the tape total are delivered to the cashier.

Upon receipt of the checks, the cashier:

- Runs an adding machine tape, which must balance with the cash journal. Should the tapes not balance, the cashier and staff person who processed the checks must review the tapes until they are in agreement.
- Alphabetizes the checks.
- Endorses the checks.
- Identifies the checks by matching each check to the appropriate account by running a patient inquiry for each payment.
- Writes on each check the patient account number and carrier/payment code.
- Prepares the bank deposit.
- Performs manual posting. Posts checks to the cash receipts journal after identification. Makes two copies of all checks; files one copy for future reference and sends the other copy to data processing for posting. Highlights the account number, name, and payment code. After posting all checks, adds and balances them to each cash receipts journal, and runs a tape total to balance with each cash receipts journal. Includes cash receipts journals from E.R., admitting, pharmacy, and so forth. Logs and batches cash receipts journals, forwards them to the Business Office Manager for approval, and submits them to data processing for keying.
- Or performs posting on-line. Posts to the appropriate account directly from the checks after identification. Files one copy of the check for future reference. The Business Office Manager verifies computerized procedures via cash posting computerized reports versus cashier's reconciliation.
- Handles any unidentified payments by first obtaining approval of the Business Office Manager, then posting payment to the Unidentified Cash Account and sending a tracer to the payor for further identification of the payment no later than the end of the next business day.
- Maintains a daily/weekly/monthly cash receipts log.

Applying Receipt and Contractual Adjustment at Time of Cash Receipt

Terminal inquiries on the accounts affected are run to verify that the computer balance is equal to the balances on the reports and also to determine what adjustment is necessary after the cash receipt has been applied.

The patient account number and general ledger number for the contractual adjustment is indicated on the remittance advice and keyed directly from the remittance advice.

The amount of the contractual adjustment is recorded as *amount withheld* along with the actual payment received. This results in the contractual adjustment being subtracted from the patient's account.

After posting, the remittance advices are forwarded to the Business Office Manager for review.

Processing Physician Payments

These payments are set up as a series or revolving account with the physician's name and address as the patient name and address, and the patient name keyed as the line description for each payment made.

A list is provided to the physician along with the hospital's check on a monthly basis.

The proper adjustment is to be made to the account (same as refund procedure) to reflect the payment to the physician, thereby clearing the credit balance on the physician's account monthly.

Lock Box System

Purpose

To ensure cash is deposited in the bank daily to maximize cash flow.

Policy

The hospital establishes a lock box system with its bank whereby mail payments are mailed directly to the bank. The bank deposits all monies the day of receipt, and sends copies of the checks received to the hospital.

Procedure

When the check copies are received, the cashier runs an adding machine tape of the check copies. If the tape does not agree with the amount deposited by the bank, the Business Office Manager must be notified immediately.

The cashier then performs all other cash posting procedures (with the exception of endorsing and depositing the checks).

Unidentified Payments

Purpose

To establish guidelines and controls for posting and applying unidentified cash.

Policy

Payments that cannot be identified the day of receipt are to be applied to an account entitled "Unidentified Cash," and deposited with other daily cash.

Procedure

When unidentified cash payments occur, the unidentified cash account number is used as the admission number for coding the cash receipts journal, and the hospital is used for guarantor name and address. Any identifying information is noted in the paid by column. A copy of the check and any other backup is kept in the file.

The unidentified account is interim billed at least monthly.

When interim bills are produced, one designated person researches the interim bill in attempt to locate accounts. The identifying information on the interim bill is in a list form, recording the information in the paid by column of the cash receipts journal.

As payments are identified, they are applied to the appropriate account by reversing the payment from the unidentified account and posting it to the legitimate account.

Unidentified payments are transferred to miscellaneous income if still unidentified after 90 days.

The Business Office Manager reviews the unidentified account regularly to determine how many dollars and how many accounts are unidentified.

Credit Balances and Refunds

Purpose

To establish standards for the prompt identification and refund of credit balance accounts receivable accounts.

Definitions

Credit Balance: An overpayment or adjustment performed on an active accounts receivable account causing the current balance to fall below zero.

Refund: A liquidation through payment of a credit balance to the source of the overpayment.

Policy

Credit balance totals should be no more than one percent of the gross accounts receivable balance and should have no accounts aged over 30 days from the date of the transaction causing the credit balance.

Procedure

A specific business office staff member is assigned responsibility to review and analyze all active accounts receivable credit balance accounts.

After review by the Business Office Manager, the credit balance listing is forwarded to the assigned staff member for processing and refund.

A refund request package is submitted to the accounting department weekly on a day determined by the accounting department and should include no less than the following:

- Refund Analysis checklist with preparer's and Business Office Manager's signatures.
- On-line inquiry documentation delineating all account activity post check-out.
- Copies of all payments posted to the account (checks, cash receipts, etc.).
- All documentation initiating account adjustment activity (Medicare allowances, courtesy discounts, etc.).

The Chief Financial Officer's approval of refunds are documented on the Refund Analysis Checklist. Administrative approval is documented by the Administrator's signature on the refund check.

To reduce the amount of paper involved, a rubber stamp that includes the information necessary for processing the refund should be used. All statistical information is available on the patient inquiry print-out, listing the payments and payors; the print-out should be stamped and completed, then submitted to accounts payable for processing.

1–31 Automated Collection Follow-up System

Purpose

To provide a method of consistent and systematic follow-up on all accounts.

Policy

Each account is to be reviewed and followed up at the appropriate time.

Procedure

All accounts on the aged trial balance are divided into equal groups using 21 days. The groups are loaded with the follow-up date, using a day of the month for each group.

Once the accounts are loaded onto the system, a follow-up report is printed daily.

The file clerk pulls the accounts listed on the follow-up report, if needed, and distributes them to the appropriate collection representative for follow-up.

When the account is worked, all documentation is entered into the system with the new follow-up date. When a patient calls or correspondence is received and new arrangements are made, or when something is done with the account that would change the expected date of payment, the new follow-up date is keyed into the system.

The biller initiates the follow-up on new accounts at the time of billing. After each account is billed, the account is documented as to the date and carrier billed, with a follow-up date of 21 days, which is keyed into the system.

Self-pay account files are documented by collections and the follow-up date keyed at the time arrangements are made, which may be at the time of admission.

All follow-up work is reviewed daily to ensure it is current and accurate.

The biller and/or the collector should review accounts demanding a higher quality of work.

1–31 Manual Collection Follow-up System

Purpose

To provide a method of consistent and systematic follow-up on all accounts.

Policy

Each account is to be reviewed and followed up at the appropriate time.

Procedure

All accounts on the aged trial balance are listed on 3 × 5 cards. The name, account number, and carrier code are the only items on the card. Multiple accounts for the same family are listed on the same card.

3 × 5 cards are made on accounts on the end of month in-house and suspense trials.

Admitting and Outpatient Registration make 3 × 5 cards on all new registrations. Each card is placed in the patient file folder.

When the insurance is billed, the follow-up date is written on the 3 × 5 card. Billing statements are reviewed by the Billing Supervisor or other designated staff, and the cards are distributed to the appropriate collectors.

For self-pay accounts, the same procedure applies, except the file is documented by collections and the card filed at the time arrangements are made, which may be during the admission.

When cards are made on all appropriate accounts, they are equally spread through the 1–31 file. This then becomes the daily collection work.

Cards for the current day are pulled and inquiries run. Any card with an account balance below $15 is thrown away. On all remaining cards, the corresponding files are pulled for follow-up.

All collection activity is documented in the actual file with the new promise-to-pay date noted. The date is also noted on the 3 × 5 card and refiled behind the corresponding day in the 1–31 file.

When a patient calls or correspondence is received and new arrangements are made, or when something is done with the account that would change the expected date of payment, the file is notated with the new promise-to-pay date and the 3 × 5 card pulled with the new date notated and refiled.

All follow-up work is reviewed daily to ensure it is done accurately and on a current basis.

Accounts needing a higher quality of work should be reviewed with employees.

The following form is used for account documentation for manual systems once the documentation area on the patient file folder is filled.

Follow-up Documentation

Date	*Documentation*

Third Party Collections

Purpose

To ensure that follow-up on every third party account is adequately and appropriately performed in a timely manner.

Policy

The following procedures represent minimum guidelines for the efficient and effective collection of third party accounts receivable. In addition, despite hospital acceptance of patient insurance assignment of benefits, the patient or guarantor is considered solely responsible for the full payment of the total charges (unless otherwise stated by legal document or power of attorney).

Procedure

Collection personnel should use the 1–31 tickler collection procedure. The file clerk pulls the folders for the accounts designated for follow-up and distributes to collectors.

Documentation of all collection work, whether received from the third party or patient or initiated by the collector, is to be maintained for all collection activity (telephone calls, interviews, letters, follow-up, tracers, etc.). Documentation should be on the account folder or in the system, as appropriate, including the following:

- Date of collection work
- Time of collection work
- Telephone number of contact
- Full name of contact
- Location of contact (work, home, patient, employer, insurance company)
- Summary of work and action taken
- Next follow-up date
- Collector's initials
- Abbreviation for most commonly used terms should be used whenever possible (see Standard Abbreviations)

Original patient financial records include the following:

- Registration form
- Itemized total charges
- Insurance claim forms, if applicable
- Any and all written correspondence
- Collection documentation

These are maintained for at least five years from date of patient discharge from the hospital. If the account has been forwarded or reported to a credit reporting agency, records should be maintained for at least seven years from date of report.

Follow-up for third party collections takes place on the assigned promise date via the 1–31 collection system.

When the account is ready for the initial follow-up and payment has not yet been received, a telephone call is made to the insurance company claims examiner to ensure the following:

- The claim has been received
- No other information is required; but if so, what kind of information (i.e., medical records), and to whom is the information to be sent?
- What expected payment amount is and when the payment will be mailed.

Once confirmation of claim receipt is obtained from the insurance claims examiner, follow-up is scheduled (not to exceed 31 days from the current contact).

If payment is not received by the follow-up date, the collector calls the claims examiner. If the date the claim was received, amount of payment, and date check will be mailed cannot be obtained, the collector should insist on speaking with the supervisor.

If the insurance company fails to honor payment of the verified claim within a reasonable time period, the insured is informed that all documentation for payment of the claim has been received by the insurance company. The insured's assistance is requested in obtaining payment from the insurance carrier.

If payment is not received from the insurance carrier within the time frame established by the hospital, the account is changed to self-pay.

When an effort has been made to collect from the patient as well as the insurance carrier and no response is received in a timely manner, the account is referred to the Business Office Manager for review.

Rejected insurance claims are changed to self-pay. The file clerk runs inquiries on the rejected account, pulls the patient file, and distributes to the appropriate collector for follow-up.

Management reviews of patient account collection files are performed daily. These reviews should include:

- Date
- Constructive analysis of work performed
- Suggestions to enhance collection activity
- Manager's initials

Managers should use a distinctive ink for reviews to differentiate reviews from routine collection documentation. A daily review is necessary by management until a comfort level is reached with the collectors, at which time a weekly review can be done from a random selection of files.

Standard Abbreviations

It is necessary that the same abbreviations be used not only on self-pay accounts but also on all other types as well, since notes made while an account is still considered third party may be crucial to its collection if and when it later becomes self-pay.

A standard form that prescribes the order in which the five (5) basic parts of most messages should be documented is shown below.

DATE	*TIME*	*WHAT OCCURRED*	*NEXT FOLLOW-UP*	*INITIALS OF PATIENT REP.*
1/7/89	13:15	Pho.Pat.Hse Spk/WP.P.B.	1/9/88	R.A.

Phoned patient house, spoke to wife, promised to pay balance 1/9/89.

Talked to—T/T	Statement—Stmt
Phoned—Pho	Weeks—Wk
Patient—Pat.	Months—Mo
Spoke—Spk	End of—EO
With—/	House—Hse
Mother—M	Job—J
Father—F	Insurance—Ins
Son—S	Blue Cross—BC
Daughter—D	Will Call Back—WCB
Mother-in-law—M—I—L	Will Be In—WBI
Promised to Pay—P.P.	Balance—B
Immediately—Imd	Return Mail—X
As Soon as Possible—ASAP	No Good—N.G.
No Answer—N/A	Bankruptcy—Bk
Left Message to Call Back—LMTCB	Disconnected—Dsct
Left No Forwarding Address—LNFA	Uncooperative—Un-Coop
Husband—H	
Wife—W	

Self-pay Collections

Purpose

To ensure that adequate and appropriate follow-up is done on every self-pay account.

Policy

Follow-up on self-pay accounts will be done consistently to ensure maximization of cash flow, and for timely identification of bad debt accounts.

Procedure

Accounts set up for payout by monthly payments should be paid timely. If a payment is not made as agreed, the collector makes one telephone call to the patient. If payment is subsequently not received, all in-house collection activity ceases and the account is referred to a collection agency.

Payment Arrangements

All accounts that require payment arrangements are set up to pay out no later than 90 days, unless approved in writing by administration.

Financial folders, with comments, for patients requiring extended payments are given to the Business Office Manager daily for review and determination.

OB Discount Package Programs

Payment for services is required to be paid in full prior to delivery due date. The Business Office Manager should approve all accounts requiring 30-day extensions.

In situations in which the patient has paid for a normal delivery but an unexpected cesarean section was performed, the facility must carefully consider its approach regarding financial requirements from the patient.

Upon discharge, final bill, and payment of services, the business office submits an adjustment for the allowance to data processing.

A series of datamailer statements are mailed to the guarantor with each message progressively stronger (if the balance remains unpaid). An initial insurance notice is mailed to patients with insurance coverage. Once the datamailers have cycled, the account is reviewed for transfer to the proper collection agency.

No telephone collection activity occurs for account balances less than $50. Computer follow-up statements are sent. If the account remains unpaid, it is referred to a pre-collect agency within 60 days, and a collection agency thereafter.

Management reviews patient account collection files daily. These reviews should include:

- Date
- Constructive analysis of work performed
- Suggestions to enhance collection activity
- Manager's initials

Managers should use a distinctive ink for reviews to differentiate reviews from routine collection documentation. A daily review is necessary by management until a comfort level is reached with the collectors, at which time a weekly review of randomly pulled files is sufficient.

Any self-pay accounts determined to be uncollectible are written off to bad debt and placed with a collection agency at the time the determination is made.

7

The Telephone Collection Call

The telephone call is a quick and relatively inexpensive method of contacting a debtor to discuss an overdue balance. It is also the most practical means of contacting other sources of information about the debtor. The telephone call is the most important collection tool.

Usually, the collector will be telephoning a patient who has not responded to collection notices and who did not, or could not, comply with the self-pay registration deposit requirement. The successful collection of the account will depend upon the collector's skill in handling that telephone call.

The procedure for telephoning an overdue account is:

- Analyze the account
- Contact the debtor at home address or place of business
- Conduct the interview

Analyzing the Account

Collectors are responsible for being well-informed about the accounts. Before telephoning the patient, review the collection memo card, folder or comments on the computer, and any media or detail attached to the file. Collectors should familiarize themselves with the patient's apparent circumstances, since a thorough knowledge of the account is necessary to discuss it intelligently with the debtor and accurately evaluate the information given. When reviewing the account, the following should be determined:

- Any payment history and the extent to which the account is past due.
- What collection effort has been expended to date with what results.
- Is the patient a chronic delinquent?
- Nature and extent of illness?

Calling the Patient

The analysis should indicate the time and the place at which the patient is most likely to be reached. When making the call, collectors should be certain they are speaking with the patient. The patient can be identified by using his or her name . . . "Is this Mr. __ ?" Only after identifying the debtor should the collector say, "I'm Mr./Ms. __ from (hospital name)." The collector pauses here for three to five seconds to allow time for a response. If the patient does not begin to discuss the account, the collector continues the conversation by stating, "I've called to talk to you about your balance with our Hospital." State the balance and the amount past due, then pause again at this point.

The Interview

During the interview, the collector is firm, but tactful, expressing confidence in the patient's integrity and intent to pay. Certain questions should be asked in order to understand the circumstances and why the balance has not been paid:

- Why is the account overdue?
- Was the patient presented all options to pay the account by cash, credit card, or special financing at the time of registration or discharge?
- Why has the patient not responded to previous collection contacts?
- Exactly when will the balance be paid? Indefinite promises such as, "I will pay next week, the middle or end of the month," are not acceptable. The promise must be pinpointed to a specific day.

- How much will be paid? The full amount due should always be requested first. Promises such as "I will pay as much as I can" are not acceptable. Partial payments, when all other options were presented at the time of registration/discharge, are unacceptable. The collector must be firm, but realistic. No purpose is served by talking persons who are working part-time making $200 per week into promising $2,000 out of their next month's pay.
- Out of what income will they pay?

  - If a patient cannot remit the full past due amount, other sources of financial assistance, such as banks, friends, or relations should be considered.
  - A patient should be reminded that paying the balance is helping to ensure that quality medical care will continue to be available for those who need it.
  - Persons who still owe a balance should *not* be told that their accounts have been closed or that they cannot come into the hospital again.

- Determine the problem with an interested, sympathetic attitude and ask intelligent questions.
- When it is necessary to obtain, update, or verify information, ask questions that require an explanation. Be a good listener. Words and manner should show genuine interest in everything the patient is saying. Control the interview. The average call should take no more than three to five minutes. For example, this approach might be used:

  "Where are you now working, Mr. ____ ?"
  "What other bills do you owe, Ms. ____ ?"

- Be objective, direct queries toward getting useful information, and be alert for new facts and changed circumstances. Take care to avoid embarrassing patients, even if their answers are inconsistent with known facts. The collector should take the "I don't understand" approach and ask for clarification.
- Ask questions specifically related to the payment of the balance to develop a solution to the problem. Be direct, but pleasant. With this approach, the collector is able to analyze each patient's situation and develop a sound basis for reaching a mutually acceptable arrangement within the ability to pay.
- Before the call is concluded, the agreement for payment or financing should be reviewed with a patient; patients must understand they are responsible for notifying the hospital if they are unable to carry out the agreement. The agreement must be documented on the file folder or in the system to ensure the patient keeps the agreement. Notes should be made during the call and the patient asked to do the same. Note-taking should not be postponed until after the call has been completed. It is wise to let the debtor know that his agreement is being written down. Do not, however, preach to or judge the patient.
- Effective handling of delinquent accounts will depend to a great extent on the collector's ability to develop good telephone technique. It is a valuable skill that can be learned with practice. Consider:

  - To the patient, the collector is the hospital. The hospital is judged by the voice that speaks over the telephone; by what is said and how it is said.
  - It is important for collectors to be certain they are talking with the patient or responsible party before discussing the account.
  - Notes should be taken during the call.
  - The collector should not indulge in unnecessary conversation, but should be friendly, courteous and businesslike.
  - Care should be taken to speak clearly so that the debtor can easily understand.
  - The person's name should be used frequently. This helps to hold his attention.
  - In concluding the call, the conversation should be terminated politely and the patient given the opportunity to hang up first.
  - Avoid expressions like "by the way," "you were sick, weren't you?" or "this is going against your credit."
  - The collector has done his job well if each call is concluded by determining how the balance will be paid and when and by keeping the goodwill of the patient.

Contact Procedure for Third Party Follow-up

Third party follow-up is also an important function of telephone collections. If the follow-up is performed appropriately, missing information required for payment can be identified quickly, and the processing and mailing of the payment can be facilitated.

When the account is ready for insurance follow-up and payment has not been received, a telephone call is made to the insurance company claims examiner to ensure the following:

- Claim has been received
- No other information is required; if so, what kind of information (i.e., medical records) and to whom is the information to be sent
- Expected payment amount and when the payment will be mailed.

When the account is ready for the next follow-up, the collector must have the file and all previous follow-up documentation before making the call.

The collector asks for the claims department and to speak with the claims examiner. If the dollar amount and date of payment cannot be obtained, insist on speaking with the supervisor. Document the first and last name of the examiner or supervisor with whom account was discussed.

- Explain the purpose of the collection call: to follow up the billing of the claim.
- The contact should be informed that the hospital has established the following policy:
  - The collector must have the date that the claim was received.
  - The collector must know when the claim will be honored and the check will be sent; not processed, but the date it will be mailed.
  - The contact should be informed that because of the outstanding balance, the file has been documented that the claim was verified and the coverage is valid.

Get assurance that all the necessary work for payment of the claim has been received from the hospital, and the claim will be processed within a set number of days. The payment is expected to be mailed to the hospital by a certain date, and receipt of the check will be documented when received.

If the insurance company fails to honor payment of the verified claim within these reasonable dates, the insured is informed that all documents for payment of their claim against their insurance company have been received by their company and verified by hospital insurance follow-up personnel. The hospital would also appreciate immediate cooperation in contacting the insurance carrier to get the matter cleared from the books.

Make clear to the insured that billing to insurance carriers is a courtesy, and prompt payment and cooperation from both insurance companies and their insureds are absolutely necessary for the hospitals to continue to provide the quality care that its patients have come to expect.

Bad Debt Write-off

Purpose

To ensure that bad debt accounts are handled consistently and appropriately.

Policy

Active patient accounts are considered bad debts when they are reviewed by the Business Office Manager and deemed uncollectible. Depending on the dollar amount of the account, the Chief Financial Officer and Administrator also review the bad debt account.

An account is generally considered uncollectible when it meets the following criteria:

- No response from the third party carrier or patient in the previous 60 days despite at least four contacts with either the responsible party or the third party carrier.
- No payment has been received and no financing could be arranged to pay the account in full in the previous 60 days despite at least four contacts with the responsible party.
- Third party carrier has denied (in writing) responsibility for any payment on the account and the collector has documented patient refusal for payment or financing.
- The account has aged 180 days without full payment.

Placement of bad debt accounts should be made monthly. Active accounts that have been reserved for bad debt should not be allowed to carry over into subsequent months with specific exception on accounts expecting full payment not to exceed four weeks.

Procedure

The collector determines the account to be uncollectible, based on established criteria.

The collector completes a transaction sheet to change the financial class to pending bad and prepares the bad debt write-off sheet, attaches both to the folder, and forwards to the Business Office Manager for review and approval.

The Business Office Manager holds all folders until the end of month.

On the 20th of the month, an accounts receivable select report is run, or the aged trial balance is used to review all accounts over 180 days for bad debt write-off.

All folders being held for write-off are matched to the list.

Depending on the amount to be written off, the Business Office Manager obtains approval for write-off from the Chief Financial Officer and Administrator.

The account is written off of active accounts receivable.

The account is placed with the appropriate collection agency.

The patient account folder is removed from the central files and stored in a separate collection agency file.

Bad Debt Write-off Sheet

The Bad Debt Write-Off Sheet is a tool to ensure that patient accounts meet the criteria required to be considered uncollectible, that all information necessary for keying the changes into the system is identified, and that all authorizations are obtained. It is not needed if appropriate policies are in place, follow-up has been according to guidelines, collectors' notes thoroughly document everything that has occurred, and the patient account folder has been signed off; however, it is an alternative approach that may be instituted.

The collector completes sections I, II, and III, attaches the sheet to the patient account file and forwards both to the Business Office Manager for review and approval. The write-off amount will determine whether additional approvals are required.

Bad Debt Placement

Purpose

To ensure that bad debt accounts are appropriately referred to collection agencies.

Policy

Placement of bad debt accounts is made monthly. Active accounts that have been reserved for bad debt should not be allowed to carry over into subsequent months with specific exception on accounts expecting full payment not to exceed four weeks.

At least two agencies will be used for referral of accounts.

Lawsuits recommended by agencies may be initiated only through the expressed written authorization of the hospital Administrator and Chief Financial Officer.

Procedure

After the account is written off active accounts receivable, it is placed with the appropriate collection agency.

Collection agency personnel should come to the hospital to make copies of the patient files. Patient files are not to leave the hospital.

Copies of patient inquiries are attached to the files.

Placement and recovery analysis reports issued monthly by collection agencies are kept in a permanent file.

Medicare Bad Debts

Purpose

To ensure that all Medicare guidelines regarding bad debt accounts are followed to maximize end-of-year Medicare reimbursement.

Definition

A debt must meet these criteria to be an allowable bad debt:

- The debt is related to covered services and derived from deductible and co-insurance amounts.
- The provider is able to establish that reasonable collection efforts were made. To be considered a reasonable collection effort, a provider's effort to collect Medicare deductible and co-insurance amounts must be similar to the effort the provider puts forth to collect comparable amounts from non-Medicare patients.
- The provider's collection effort is documented in the patient's file by copies of bills, follow-up letters, reports of telephone and personal contacts, collection agency acknowledgment and return.

Policy

Medicare accounts determined to be bad debts must meet Medicare criteria and have reasonable collection efforts to be reimbursed on the end-of-year cost report.

If, after reasonable and customary attempts to collect a bill, a debt remains unpaid more than 120 days from the date the first bill is mailed to the beneficiary, the account may be written off to bad debt and referred to an agency unless it is considered charity.

Bad Debt Write-off Sheet

Patient Name ______________________________ Acct # ______________________

Bad Debt Financial Class __________ Trans Code ______________________

I. Criteria for Write-off:

_____ Patient uncooperative

_____ Lien filed

_____ Unsuccessful phone attempt

_____ Broken payment promise

$ __________ Amt past due

__________ # months past due

_____ No valid information from phone, friends, references

_____ No response to final notice

_____ Evidence of loan denial attached

_____ No response to phone contact

_____ Financial statement completed

_____ Insurance company uncooperative

_____ Bankruptcy notice received __________

_____ Mail return, unsuccessful skip

_____ No alternative payment source

_____ Other (Explain) ____

II. Type of Account:

_____ Original self-pay

_____ Balance after Medicare

_____ Balance after insurance

_____ Balance after HMO/PPO contract

_____ Worker's comp denied

_____ Outpatient _____ Inpatient

III. Recommended Action:

What would you estimate is the probability that this account will be recovered by an outside agency?

_____ Good _____ Fair _____ Poor

_____ Assign to agency

_____ Age of account at write-off

_____ Bankrupt

_____ Recommended write-off $ __________

_____ Administrative write-off

_____ Legal/Lien/Creditor's claim

Date Filed __________

_____ Uncollectible. Why? ____

Prepared by: ______________________________ Date ______________

IV. Approval:

Amount	Title	Signature	Date
To $1000	Business Office Manager	____________	______
$1000–$5000	Chief Financial Officer	____________	______
$5000+	Administrator	____________	______

V. Instructions: Complete sections I, II, & III. Attach to jacket and refer to supervisor for review and approval.

Procedure

Account is written off to a collection agency.

Account information will be logged on the Medicare Bad Debt Log:

- Patient name
- HIB number
- Dates of service(s)
- Bad debt amount

To substantiate a bad debt amount, remittance advice information must be posted to the log:

- Remittance advice date
- Deductible amount
- Co-insurance amount
- Non-covered amount (although this amount is not reimbursable, it will show what portion of bills are deemed bad debt)

If the entire bad debt amount is non-covered, there will be no need to log account.

Any future payments will be entered on the log.

Since uncollected amounts are reimbursable at year-end, the Business Office Manager must verify all accounts listed on the log that have not been collected. If an account has been paid out, a line is drawn across the information so that it will not be included in the totals.

All logs are forwarded to the Chief Financial Officer to be entered on the cost report.

Medicare Denials

Purpose

To ensure that all Medicare denials are handled consistently and appropriately.

Policy

In the event a Medicare inpatient bill is denied by the Peer Review Organization (PRO), the U.R. Coordinator will keep the Business Office Manager aware of any appeals and the findings on each denial. If an account is not eligible for the appeal process, the U.R. Coordinator will notify the Business Office Manager in writing and such notification will be placed in the patient file.

Accounts receivable will be adjusted to accurately reflect the denial.

Procedure

Denied accounts are logged separately on the Medicare Bad Debt Log for the Business Office Manager to follow up on the status of the appeals process with the U.R. Coordinator.

A copy of the denial is placed in the patient folder and the account is written off as a PRO denial to an allowance account.

If the facility is PIPing Medicare, and denials are received on accounts that have been PIPed off the active accounts receivable, the accounts should be reactivated and ancillary services billed to Part B. When the PIP is retracted and Part B charges have been paid, the balance of the account is written off as a PRO denial.

Incoming Correspondence

Purpose

To establish controls to ensure consistent and timely resolution of incoming correspondence.

Policy

All correspondence is to be opened, logged according to types of problems, distributed, and worked on a timely, consistent basis.

Procedure

Correspondence is opened and logged on the Correspondence Log daily according to the nature of the problems.

Pre-authorizations, pre-certifications, approvals, referrals are pulled; patient inquiries are run to determine if patient is in-house or discharged.

Corresponding authorization for pre-admissions and in-house accounts is taken to Admitting for filing in the appropriate patient file.

Pre-authorizations for discharged accounts are filed in the appropriate account in the business office. Location of the account should be the pending file in billing, awaiting the same document.

The balance of the correspondence is placed in the basket for the file clerks to pull.

File clerks pull the corresponding file, run a patient inquiry, and turn the account over to the collector or designated person other than the billers to work.

The following form is used to determine the trends of incoming correspondence and assists the Business Office Manager in knowing if the correspondence is legitimate or is actually being created by the hospital employees.

Correspondence Log

Ins. Req. Info = Insurance requested information
Need Int. Bill = Need Interim Bill
Adt Req. = Audit Request   Adt Res. = Audit Results
Pr-Au Certs = Pre-authorization Certs
Ins. Den. = Insurance Denial   Ml Ret. = Mail Return
Clm Ret. = Claim Return   Aty Req. = Attorney Request

Date	Ins. Req. Info	Need Int. Bill	Adt Req.	Adt Res.	Pr-Au Certs	Ins. Den.	Ml Ret.	Clm Ret.	Aty Req.	Other

Correspondence is to be worked to a conclusion daily and the collection notes dated and documented as to action taken.

Any correspondence that is forwarded, e.g., request for medical records, is copied and placed in the patient file with appropriate documentation in the collection notes.

All correspondence not completed by Friday is referred to the Business Office Manager for evaluation.

The Correspondence Log is given to the Business Office Manager weekly for review.

Third Party Audits

Purpose

To provide guidelines for proper protection of confidential patient information and prompt payment of audited accounts, and to improve billing accuracy.

Policy

Third party audit firms must notify the hospital in writing of an intended audit and set up an appointment to perform the audit. Payment of 80 percent of the account balance should be made by the time of the audit. Payment of the audit fee for administrative time should be made at the time of the audit.

Procedure

The request for an audit is presented in writing to the hospital. Include the following information in the audit request letter:

- Name of patient whose account is to be audited
- Patient account number
- Dates of service
- Reason the claim was selected for audit
- Duly authorized patient consent (in the instance of a minor, deceased patient, or patient unable to sign, the notarized signature of a properly authorized representative with a statement of relationship to the patient will be accepted)
- Name of the insurance carrier or other third party who requested the audit
- Name of the firm and name of the individual (if known) who will perform the audit

Upon receipt of the letter, the Quality Assurance Coordinator (or other designated staff person) confirms the receipt of the required information, determines that the third party payor has satisfied in full its contractual payment obligation with its subscriber, and schedules an appointment date with the auditor.

Undercharges as well as overcharges are addressed on all audits, and all departments where discrepancies are found are involved in the audit.

Charges for all questioned documentation are interpreted by utilizing hospital medical records, departmental logs, and qualified medical expertise.

Audits are limited to verifying that the charges on the detail bill were for services rendered and the charges are accurate. No discussions are held with any third party auditor regarding the reasonableness of any charge, nor will any financial data or reports regarding pricing policies of the hospital be disclosed.

Questions regarding medical necessity of the services provided are considered separately from the billing audit. Hospital approved services provided are billable to the patient with or without recorded physician orders.

Upon completion of the audit, an exit conference is held. No audit results are accepted unless agreed on by the hospital auditor and the insurance auditor. The confirmation of adjustment letter is to be signed by both auditors, verifying the adjusted balance.

After the exit conference, the adjustments are submitted to the business office for rebilling. In an instance of overcharge, the hospital issues a refund promptly upon receipt of request for refund. If underpaid, the hospital will expect prompt payment to be issued for its rebilled claim.

Failure of the third party to agree to this policy precludes the third party from gaining access to the medical record and detail bill.

A copy of this policy should be forwarded to medical records.

Patient Account Filing

Purpose

To establish a system for pulling and refiling patient account files so accounts can be located at all times.

Policy

Patient account files are to be filed by the file clerks in complete alphabetical sequence within each patient surname.

Procedure

File clerks are responsible for pulling and refiling all patient files in the appropriate area: open, closed, or bad debt files. The only exception is when a file is needed immediately for a patient telephone call. The person taking the call is allowed to retrieve the file if a message cannot be taken; however, it is to be refiled by the file clerk.

Each employee appropriately documents the file to indicate open, closed, bad debt, collection agency status, etc. Final responsibility is with the file clerk to assure file status is documented.

Employees requesting patient account files submit a list to the file clerks. The file clerks pull the charts and replace them with the appropriate outcard for files leaving the business office area. Outcards are not necessary for files remaining in the business office.

Departments requesting files will place a "File Request" form in the file request box. Each department should turn in its requests to the file clerk no later than 3:00 P.M. for pickup the next morning.

The file clerks pull all charts during the last two hours of their working day.

In the case of a special chart request or a single chart request, the file clerks pull that chart immediately and present it to the requesting party.

Returned files are placed on the "file back" shelves. The file clerks refile the charts.

Collection agency stamps take precedence over an account with a zero written on it. The zero should be crossed off.

The zero statement provides all activity ever posted to the patient account after discharge and is filed in each individual patient's folder.

It is the file clerk's responsibility to notify the Business Officer Manager of all unlocated files no later than Friday of each week.

8

Bankruptcy Collections*

Purpose

To provide basic information and guidance for handling a patient account on notification of the patient's bankruptcy.

How a Bankruptcy Proceeding Begins

When a patient becomes insolvent, the patient ("debtor") may obtain the protection of the bankruptcy code by filing a petition in bankruptcy court. This is known as a voluntary filing. Alternatively, creditors of an insolvent debtor may file such a petition. This is called an involuntary filing. In either case, the bankruptcy court immediately issues a document called an order for relief. The petition and order essentially begin the bankruptcy proceedings and are generally used as the starting points from which the court measures important time limits. Shortly after the court issues the order for relief, the court or the debtor notifies all creditors of the debtor of the pending bankruptcy proceeding.

What Action to Take

The bankruptcy petition operates as a court order that prohibits virtually all collection efforts against the debtor while the bankruptcy proceeding remains pending. This attribute of the petition is known as the automatic stay. Once the petition is filed, all creditors, including the hospital and its agents, must cease all collection efforts in progress and refrain from instituting any new efforts. This means that the hospital must not file or continue to prosecute any suit against the debtor, send a bill or statement to the debtor, refer the matter to a collection agent, or take any other similar action. If the hospital previously referred the matter to a collection agent, the hospital must inform that agent of the pending bankruptcy proceeding and instruct the agent to cease all collection efforts. Bankruptcy courts zealously enforce the stay and treat violations of it very seriously. Creditors who knowingly violate the stay are often forced to pay compensatory and punitive damages to the debtor.

The one action that creditors, including the hospital, may take without violating the stay, indeed the one action that creditors generally should take, is to file a proof of claim in bankruptcy court. A proof of claim is an itemized statement indicating how the debtor became indebted to the creditor and the current amount of the unpaid debt. A photocopy of the patient's itemized bill, accompanied by a completed and signed proof-of-claim form, will normally suffice. The notice of a bankruptcy filing that a hospital receives will normally indicate where the hospital must file its proof of claim. The hospital should submit its proof of claim to the clerk of the bankruptcy court in duplicate, along with a cover letter requesting the clerk to file the original proof of claim and to return the copy to the hospital after stamping it with the time and date of filing. The hospital should also request a copy of all future notices concerning the proceeding.

The notice of a bankruptcy filing that the hospital receives will also normally set a date for a meeting of creditors and possibly for a financial examination of the debtor. Attendance at this meeting is not required, and

*The publishers appreciate the gracious assistance of Stephen L. Sepinuck, Visiting Assistant Professor of Law at IIT Chicago–Kent College of Law, in the preparation of this chapter.

the hospital personnel normally do not appear unless specifically requested to do so by the bankruptcy judge or the debtor's attorney or unless the debtor's unpaid account with the hospital is abnormally large. In most bankruptcy proceedings involving individuals (Chapter 7 and Chapter 13 proceedings), the hospital must file its proof of claim within 90 days after the first date set for the creditors' meeting.

After receiving notice of a patient's bankruptcy filing, hospitals may wish to remove the patient's account from its list of active receivables. However, the filing of a bankruptcy petition does not necessarily mean that payment will never be made or even that payment is unlikely. A hospital should confer with its accountant or tax attorney as to when such an account should be removed.

Bankruptcy Proceedings

The bankruptcy code now permits individuals to invoke any of four different bankruptcy proceedings, each generally known and referred to by the separate part of the code that governs it: Chapter 7, Chapter 11, Chapter 12, and Chapter 13.

A Chapter 7 proceeding is a liquidation. After the court issues the order for relief in a Chapter 7 proceeding, it usually appoints a trustee to act as a guardian of the debtor's property. The trustee represents the creditors with unsecured claims. As part of this representation, the trustee investigates the financial affairs of the debtor, liquidates the debtor's property as quickly as possible, makes a detailed report to the court of all transactions, and, pursuant to court direction, distributes assets to creditors.

The remaining three types of proceedings provide for various types of reorganizations. An individual who does not file a liquidation petition under Chapter 7, and who has a regular source of income, will most probably file for reorganization under Chapter 13 (Chapter 11 is also available to individuals, although some courts restrict it to those who operate a business; Chapter 12 is available to family farmers). In Chapter 13 proceedings, as in all reorganizations, the debtor remains in control of all of the debtor's assets (the "bankruptcy estate"). If the court appoints a trustee, the trustee merely oversees the debtor's administration of the bankruptcy estate. The debtor then seeks to use the assets of the estate to generate sufficient income to pay off the creditors pursuant to a plan of reorganization. The bankruptcy code gives the debtor the exclusive right to file a plan of reorganization in Chapter 13 proceedings. In Chapter 11 proceedings, this exclusive right exists only for the 120 days immediately following the order for relief; after that time, creditors may propose alternative plans.

Each proposed plan of reorganization divides creditors into various groups and details when and what proportion of their claims the debtor will pay each group. The rules regarding the content and approval of plans are varied and complex. Suffice it to say that the bankruptcy court, after a hearing, will approve one plan. Once the court approves a plan of reorganization, a process called "confirmation," the debtor will attempt to comply with the plan. In the event circumstances change significantly, either the debtor or a creditor may seek a change in the plan. Once the debtor makes all the payments called for in the plan (as finally approved and modified) or liquidates under Chapter 7, the court will issue an order discharging the debtor of most debts that arose before the original bankruptcy filing. This order prohibits creditors from collecting or attempting to collect any discharged debt. The hospital must not seek to enforce or otherwise try to collect a discharged debt. Any attempt to do so may place the hospital in contempt of court and subject it to serious penalties.

Terms Used in Bankruptcy Cases

Bankruptcy Estate

The bankruptcy estate consists of all of the debtor's property and assets at the time the bankruptcy petition is filed, together with certain property and assets acquired by the debtor or the trustee after the bankruptcy filing.

Chapter 11

Laymen often describe any petition for bankruptcy relief as "filing Chapter 11." The reasons for this rest in the historical meaning and usage of the term. Under the modern bankruptcy code, however, Chapter 11 is in reality only one of several different types of bankruptcy proceedings.

Creditors' Committee

Creditors of the debtor with unsecured claims may form a committee to consult with, advise, and make recommendations to the trustee with respect to the administration of the bankruptcy estate.

Discharge

A discharge is an order of the bankruptcy court that releases the debtor from the obligation to pay most of the debts owed at the time the bankruptcy petition was filed. Certain debts cannot be discharged. In addition, a debtor who has received a discharge within the last six years is not eligible for a discharge in a Chapter 7 liquidation proceeding.

Priorities

Certain expenses and claims must be paid in full before any payment is made to creditors on general unsecured claims. These special expenses and claims are called priorities. The most common priorities are these: (1) the costs of administering the bankruptcy proceeding, including the trustee's fee; (2) wages earned by, but not paid to, employees of the debtor within 90 days before the filing of the petition; and (3) most federal and state taxes.

Proof of Claim

A proof of claim is a statement filed by a creditor that declares and documents the amount and nature of the debt that the debtor owes the creditor. A creditor must file a proof of claim in most bankruptcy proceedings in order to share in the assets of the bankruptcy estate. A creditor need not file a proof of claim in a Chapter 11 proceeding if that claim is included in the debtor's schedule of liabilities and is not listed there as disputed, contingent, or unliquidated.

Secured Claim

A secured claim is one for which the creditor has a security interest or lien in certain property of the debtor. The property secured may be real estate, as with a mortgage, or may be almost any type of personal property.

Trustee

A trustee is a person appointed by the bankruptcy court to take legal title to the debtor's property, administer and eventually sell the assets in the bankruptcy estate, and, on the order of the court, distribute the proceeds of those assets to the creditors. A trustee represents the collective interests of the unsecured claimholders. A trustee does not represent the interests of any single creditor with an unsecured claim or the interests of any creditor with a secured claim.

Unsecured Claim

An unsecured claim is either a debt for which the creditor holds no security interest or the portion of a secured debt that exceeds the value of the security. A general unsecured claim is an unsecured claim that is not entitled to any priority. Most hospital accounts are general unsecured claims.

9

Accounts Receivable Reporting

Reports can provide valuable tools in the management of accounts receivable.

Purpose

To evaluate A/R performance, compare performance to standards, and determine trends and identify potential problem areas on a timely basis.

Definitions

A/R Indicators—Aspects of accounts receivable (cash, billing, collections, etc.) comprising basic standards for measuring progression and/or regression in accounts receivable totals.

A/R Analysis—Used to determine trends in A/R indicators and isolate existing potential problem areas.

Statistical Analysis—Used to compare performance to standards and acceptable ranges.

Policy

The Business Office Manager completes the appropriate management reports timely and consistently, and forwards reports to the Chief Financial Officer and Administrator for their review.

Procedure

A/R Weekly Reports

The hospital Business Office Manager uses standard daily monitoring reports for all departments of the hospital business office to accurately measure performance in the following areas:

Registration
- Collections
- Number of registrations:
  - Pre-registration
  - Walk-in (non-emergency)
  - Direct
  - Emergency room (acute care only)

Cash Flow
- Charge-Based Cash
- Cost-Based Cash
- Charge-Based Revenue
- Cost-Based Revenue

Insurance Billing
- Billed Claims
- Unbilled Claims

Collection performance

Automated Report Management
- Any exception reports
- Credit balance
- Minimum balance
- Daily exceptions
- Accounts receivable total

The daily monitoring reports are recapped by the hospital Business Office Manager weekly and at month-end with copies to the Hospital Chief Financial Officer and Administrator.

A/R Monthly Reports

The Business Office Manager is responsible for completing the A/R analysis monthly. The Chief Financial Officer ensures it is accurately completed. The Business Office Manager should be trained and knowledgeable in the accurate completion and interpretation of the A/R analysis and A/R days calculation.

All A/R analysis criteria are measured against standards to achieve ideal days in A/R by using the A/R indicator report and acceptable ranges each month to evaluate performance.

A statistical analysis of the A/R analysis should be performed each month.

The Chief Financial Officer is responsible for training the Business Office Manager in completion and accuracy of the A/R analysis each month.

A/R Analysis

1. *Days in A/R Gross*

Previous month total revenue	= (+) ______	No. of Days	= (+) ______
Prior month total revenue	= (+) ______	No. of Days	= (+) ______
Current month total revenue	= (+) ______	No. of Days	= (+) ______
Total 3-month revenue	= ______	Total Days	= ______

Total 3 months revenue		______
Divided by no. of days in period	÷	______
Equals average revenue per day	=	______
Total current mo. receivable (from G/L)	=	______
Divided by average revenue per day	÷	______
Equals gross A/R days	=	______

2. *Collections per Day* (charge-based and cost-based)—the Business Office Manager keeps daily cash flow records on total dollars collected on patient account receivables during the current month, excluding rental and other income items not related to patient account receivables. Statistics are separated by charge- and cost-based payors so average cash per day may be properly calculated by payor.

3. *Average Net Revenue per Day*—Net Patient Revenue for the current month divided by the number of days in the current month.

4&5. *Billing Suspense Days* (inpatient and outpatient)—These figures should be completed with the values documented on the A/R profile at the end of the current month and should not include goals or intended reductions.

6&7. *Total Inpatient* (amount and number)

	No.	*AMOUNT*
Total Active (ATB) =	(+) ______	(+) ______
Total Cr. Bal. (ATB) =	(+) ______	(+) ______
Total Unapplied Cash =	(+) ______	(+) ______
Total In-house (I/H & Susp Listing)	(+) ______	(+) ______
Total Susp (I/H Susp Listing)	(+) ______	(+) ______
Total Inpatient	______	______

8&9. *Total Outpatient* (amount and number)

		No.		*AMOUNT*
Total Active (ATB) =	(+)	________	(+)	________
Total Cr. Bal. (ATB) =	(+)	________	(+)	________
Total Unapplied Cash =	(+)	________	(+)	________
Total Suspense (I/H & Susp Listing)	(+)	________	(+)	________
Total Outpatient =		________		________

10&11. *Credit Balances* (amount and number)—Use the prior week's credit balance listing and subtract the number and dollar amount *refunded* prior to month-end post printing of the final credit balance listing.

12. *In-house and Suspense $$*—Use the total amount documented on the month-end total aging.

13. *Aging of Discharged Accounts*—Use the appropriate aged trial balance computer report.

14. *0–90* (exclude in-house)

		AMOUNT
Total third party IP	(+)	________
Total third party OP	(+)	________
Total self-pay IP	(+)	________
Total self-pay OP	(+)	________
Less excess IP (if applicable)	(−)	________
Less excess OP (if applicable)	(−)	________
TOTAL 0–90 .... ________		

15. *91–180* (no in-house included)

		AMOUNT
Net Total A/R	(+)	________
Plus Credit Balances	(+)	________
TOTAL 91–180		________

16. *Over 180* (no in-house included)

		AMOUNT
Net Total A/R	(+)	________
Plus Credit Balances	(+)	________
TOTAL over 180		________

Please Note: (Line 12 + Line 14 + Line 15 + Line 16) = (Line 6 + Line 8). These categories *must* balance to ensure proper reporting.

17. *Under 180 Less M/M*

Line 12	(+)	________
Line 14	(+)	________
Line 15	(+)	________
Less I/P Medicare Carrier net total (after excess) =	(−)	________
Less I/P Medicaid Carrier net total (after excess) =	(−)	________
	=	________ Total under 180 Less M/M

18. *Over 180 Less M/M*

Line 16 =	(+)	________
Less I/P Medicare Carrier Net Total (after excess) =	(−)	________
Less I/P Medicaid Carrier, Net Total (after excess) =	(−)	________
	=	________ Total Over 180 Less M/M

Please Note: (Line 17 + Line 18) = (Line 1 on Days of Revenue in Accounts Receivable Calculation). This reconciliation ensures that the general ledger gross charge-based receivable is in balance with the detailed accounts receivable figures.

19. *Unbilled Insurance Amount*—This figure is best calculated by a manual summation of total dollars pending billing on the evening of the last day of the month.

20. *Total Write-Offs*

21–29. *Bad Debts*—These figures are best derived from manual record-keeping by the Business Office Manager, if the computer system will not calculate.

30. *Days Revenue Unbilled*

In-house and Suspense (Line 12)	= (+)	________
Unbilled Insurance Amt. (Line 19)	= (+)	________
Total Unbilled	=	________

Divided by Avg. Net Revenue Per Day ________ = ________ Days Revenue Unbilled

31. *% Receivables Collected*

Collections per Day (Line 2)	=	________
Times No. of Calendar Days in Cur. Mo.	(×)	________
Total Current Receivables Collected =	(+)	________
Plus Total Inpatient Amount (Line 6) =	(+)	________
Plus Total Outpatient Amt. (Line 8) =	(+)	________
Total Receivables		________

Total Cur. Receivables Collected = ________

Divided by Total Receivables = ________ = ________ % Receivable Collected

A/R Analysis

Month Ended ____________________

($ IN THOUSANDS)

		MONTH		1	2	3	4	5	6	7	8	9	10	11	12
1		Days in A/R-Gross													
2		Collections per Day													
3		Avg. Net Revenue per Day													
		Billing													
4		Suspense	Inpatient												
5		Days	Outpatient												
	A	Total Inpatient:													
6	C		Amount												
7	C		Number												
	T	Total Outpatient:													
8	S		Amount												
9			Number												
	R	Credit Balances:													
10	E		Amount												
11	C		Number												
12	E	Inhouse & Suspense $													
13	I	Aging of Dischg. Accts.													
14	V		0–90												
15	A		91–180												

($ IN THOUSANDS)

	MONTH		1	2	3	4	5	6	7	8	9	10	11	12
16	B	Over 180												
17	L	Under 180 less M/M												
18	E	Over 180 less M/M												
19		Unbilled Ins. Amount												
20		Total Write-Offs												
21	B	Agency Referrals												
	A	(name)												
22	D	1												
23		2												
24	D	3												
25	E	Agency Recoveries												
26	B	1 Fee %												
27	T	2 Fee %												
28	S	3 Fee %												
29		Total Fees Paid to Agencies												
30	Days Revenue Unbilled													
31	% Receivables Collected													

Statistical Analysis

Month Ending ________________

Collections per Day—This amount should be equal to or greater than net revenue per day. If collections per day are less than 97% of net revenue per day for any two out of four months, corrective action is necessary.

A/R Analysis

(4 mos. including current)

Month	*Yr.*		*Collect/Day*		*Net Rev/Day*			*Standard*
______	/	=		/		=	______ %	100%
______	/	=		/		=	______ %	100%
______	/	=		/		=	______ %	100%
______	/	=		/		=	______ %	100%

Billing Suspense Days—I/P and O/P suspense days should be no higher than three.

Current	*Standard*
I/P =	I/P = 3
O/P =	O/P = 3

Total Number of Inpatient Accounts—This number should never be higher than 2.5 times average monthly inpatient discharges. If this figure is higher than the standard, accounts are neither collected nor written off in a timely manner.

Current			*Standard*		
Total Active IP (ATB)	+	__________	Avg. No. Disch	=	__________
Misapplied Pmts. (ATB−IP)	+	__________			× 2.5
Total In-house (IH & Susp)	+	__________		=	__________
Total Susp (IH & Susp)	+	__________			
Total IP		__________			

Total Number of Outpatient Accounts—This figure should not be over 1.5 times the number of ER and OP visits. If this figure is larger than the standard, accounts are neither being collected nor written off in a timely manner.

Current			*Standard*		
Total Active OP (ATB) (incl. series)	+	__________	Total OP/ER Visits	=	__________
Misapplied Pmts. (ATB)	+	__________			× 1.5
Total Suspense	+	__________			
Total OP		__________		=	__________

Credit Balances—This figure should be no more than 1 percent of net accounts receivable. The goal should be set for zero credit balances and the listing cleared weekly thereafter. Timely refunds promote good public relations and a reduction of present A/R.

Current	*Standard*
#: ________	#: ________
$: ________	$: ________
________ % of Total A/R	________ % of Total A/R

In-House and Suspense—This number should be no more than average length of stay plus three multiplied by the average daily gross patient revenue. A current figure larger than the standard indicates a lack of in-house self-pay collection.

Current		*Standard*	
________	= Total Amount from A/R IH & Susp. List	________	(Avg. LOS)
		+ 3	
			× (Avg. Daily GIR)
		= ________	

Aging

	Current Stat	*% of Total*	*Standard*	*% of Total*
0–90 =		%		84%
91–180 =		%		13%
181–Over =	________	%		3%
	________	100%	________	100%

0–90 days —should be an average of 84% of gross A/R
90–180 days —should be an average of 13% of gross A/R
181 and over —should be an average of 3% of gross A/R

Bad Debts—Bad debts should be no higher than 2.5–3.75 percent of revenue. If this figure is higher than the standard, accounts are not being written off in a timely manner.

Current		*Standard*
YTD Provision for Doubtful Accts.	________	2.5–3.75%
% of Gross Patient Revenue	________	

Days in Accounts Receivables—Gross

To calculate gross days in accounts receivable, the total revenue per month and number of days in each month for the prior three months are totaled. The total three months' revenue is divided by the total number of days to arrive at an average daily revenue. The current gross receivables are then divided by the average daily revenue to determine current gross days in accounts receivable.

EXAMPLE:

MONTH	*DAYS*	*REVENUE*
January	31	2,515,000
February	29	2,483,000
March	31	2,583,000
TOTAL	91	7,581,000 = 83,308 Average Per Day

$$\frac{\text{3,903,000 Gross Receivables}}{\text{83,308 Average Revenue Per Day}} = \text{46.9 Gross Days in Receivables}$$

_____ Administrator Copied
_____ Controller Copied
_____ Corporate Copied
_____ Bus. Off. Mgr. Copied

HOSPITAL NAME ____

A/R Weekly Activity and Assessment

Registration (Standard is 30 minutes for complete admission process with verification per admission, 15 minutes without verification, and 10 minutes for E. R. admission without verification.)

Number of admissions and/or OP, ER Registrations by individual:

			TOTAL
Shift ( ) ____	Shift ( ) ____	Shift ( ) ____	________
Shift ( ) ____	Shift ( ) ____	Shift ( ) ____	________
Shift ( ) ____	Shift ( ) ____	Shift ( ) ____	________
Shift ( ) ____	Shift ( ) ____	Shift ( ) ____	________

COMMENTS ____

Number of employee productivity reports reviewed (total employees × seven workdays = __________)
Reviewed __________

COMMENTS ____

Billing (Standard is 50 claims minimum per day per biller—equivalent, nine minutes per claim—gradually increasing to 70–80 claims.)

Number and amount of claims billed per biller:

	NUMBER	AMOUNT
Full Time Biller #1	________	________
Full Time Biller #2	________	________
Full Time Biller #3	________	________
Full Time Biller #4	________	________
Total of Part Time Billers	________	________
Total Claims Billed	________	________
Combined Weekly Standard	________	________

COMMENTS ____

____

____

____

Number and amount of all claims including ER and OP unbilled:

	NUMBER	AMOUNT
Pending Medicare—Attestations	________	________
Pending Diagnosis	________	________
Pending Coding	________	________
Pending Blue Cross Approvals	________	________
Ready to Bill	________	________
Other	________	________
Total	________	________

COMMENTS ____

____

____

____

Accounts Receivable

General Ledger Posting Summary Month-to-Date:

REVENUE	ADJUSTMENTS	PAYMENTS	NET CHANGE
________	________	________	________

General Ledger Posting Summary Month End Totals:

REVENUE	ADJUSTMENTS	PAYMENTS	NET CHANGE
________	________	________	________

COMMENTS: ____

____

____

____

Total follow-up by Collector on all types of accounts (Standard is 40 contacts per day per person—Equivalent: 1 contact every 11 minutes)

	NUMBER	AMOUNT
Collector #1	______	______
Collector #2	______	______
Collector #3	______	______
Collector #4	______	______
Other	______	______
Total	______	______
Combined Weekly Standard	______	______

COMMENTS: ______________________________
____
____
____

Number of follow-up accounts collection notes reviewed ______________________________

General

	NUMBER	AMOUNT
Number and amount of credit balances:	______	______

COMMENTS ______________________________
____
____
____

	NUMBER
Number of admission files reviewed requiring corrections:	______

COMMENTS ______________________________
____
____
____

	NUMBER	AMOUNT
Number and amount of misapplied payments, adjustments, or charges:	______	______

COMMENTS ______________________________
____
____
____

	NUMBER
Number of insurance rejections:	______

COMMENTS ______________________________

____

____

____

	NUMBER	AMOUNT
Number and amount of Unidentified Cash:	______	______

COMMENTS ______________________________

____

____

____

	NUMBER	AMOUNT
Number and amount of Late Charges:	______	______

COMMENTS ______________________________

____

____

____

	NUMBER	AMOUNT
Number and amount of Accounts Receivable:	______	______

COMMENTS ______________________________

____

____

____

	AMOUNT
Amount of computer downtime:	______

COMMENTS ______________________________

____

____

____

All logging and posting of remittance advices are current through what date? ______________

COMMENTS ______________________________

____

____

____

AMOUNT

How many pieces of correspondence, including mail returns, remain unworked? ________

COMMENTS ____
____
____
____

Is your filing current? ______ Yes ______ No

COMMENTS ____
____
____
____

A

Business Office Job Descriptions and Standards of Performance

A job description must define the responsibilities and authority to achieve the expected results or conditions of a job. Standards of performance are those expected results, or conditions that do or do not come about as a result of defining one's responsibilities and authority to carry them out.

Just as important as having job descriptions in writing is ascertaining that these responsibilities, authority, and standards are discussed and explained to the employee. Staff specialists, while visiting many hospitals, hear employees voice their number one complaint, "I don't know where I stand." This usually indicates employees who do not know what their responsibilities are, what authority they have to "get things done," and when and if they have done an acceptable or unacceptable job. It is important that the Business Office Manager develop job descriptions for each employee. Individual employees should not be expected to fill out their job descriptions as far as defining responsibilities and goals. Once defined and accepted by hospital management, these responsibilities and standards should be discussed with the employee. The employee should be asked to play an active part in setting realistic standards of performance or goals.

It should be a responsibility and standard for the Business Office Manager to consistently review employee performances and ascertain that each employee knows, at all times, how he or she is measuring up to defined standards. Standards should be evaluated regularly to make sure they are realistic and achievable. Standards should be accurately matched with responsibilities. As an example: it would not be realistic to expect a collector to be responsible for achieving registration deposits on at least 60 percent of inpatients when the collector is not normally involved in the registration function.

The following job descriptions outline each business office responsibility.

Business Office Manager

Identification

Title: Business Office Manager

Department: Business Office

Supervisor: Chief Financial Officer

Position Description

Position Summary

Responsible for managing accounts receivable. Responsible for the activities of inpatient, outpatient, and emergency room registration, switchboard, cashiering, billing, and credit and collections. Coordinates operations with other hospital units and medical staff. Interprets policies and recommends policy changes to Chief Financial Officer. Interviews and hires new employees and assigns them to various work areas.

Duties and Responsibilities

Responsible for the timely billing and collection of patient charges.

Monitors bad debt and contractual losses against budgeted levels.

Monitors compliance with hospital and administration policies and directives.

Coordinates operations through direction of area supervisors.

Supervises the preparation and maintenance of departmental policy and procedure manuals.

Conducts regular periodic staff meetings to inform staff of changes in policies and to provide in-service training.

Establishes controls and review mechanisms for every procedure to ensure that systems and procedures are being followed correctly.

Develops specific objectives, budgets, and performance standards for each area of responsibility.

Monitors progress for each area on a daily basis, utilizing quantitative productivity reports.

Prepares A/R weekly and monthly reports and bad debt projections for Chief Financial Officer.

Reviews write-off listings, refund requests, miscellaneous cash adjustments, and departmental expense vouchers and submits to administration for approval.

Reviews all remittance advices; determines significant problems causing rejections and denials.

Reviews all incoming correspondence to determine problem areas.

Communicates new procedures to other hospital departments.

Resolves patient, physician, and interdepartmental complaints and misunderstandings.

Communicates with third party payors in regards to claim processing difficulties or new processing procedures.

Reviews all collection files and daily follow-up work and discusses any discrepancies with appropriate employee.

Reviews a random sampling of insurance billings on a routine basis to ensure claims are billed correctly and sent to proper mailing addresses.

Reviews admission and registration files after the Director of Admissions to ensure all information is correctly obtained.

Reviews all employees' work on a periodic basis.

Qualifications

Graduation from a recognized college or university with a degree in business administration or related area is desirable.

Two years' experience in a similar position within a hospital or related field is required.

Participation in special workshops or training sessions in Medicare, Medicaid, and Blue Cross procedures to maintain current knowledge relative to these procedures.

Knowledge of and experience with automated systems required.

Assistant Business Office Manager

Identification

Title: Assistant Business Office Manager

Department: Business Office

Supervisor: Business Office Manager

Position Description

Position Summary

An overall responsibility for submission of claims on a timely basis, rebilling, logging functions, and determination of collectibility of all patient accounts.

Duties and Responsibilities

Supervises third party claims submission.

Supervises and maintains follow-up procedures on a timely basis.

Trains new employees and holds in-house training sessions.

Maintains diagnosis follow-up procedure and working relationship with Medical Records Director.

Maintains daily billing and collections productivity reports.

Reviews in-house patient listing daily and directs interim billing in accordance with hospital procedures.

Supervises logging procedures and ascertains that logs are current at all times.

Supervises handling of inquiries from carriers and patients regarding insurance claims and ascertains that they are answered correctly and timely.

Supervises timely preparation of input documents and submission to data processing.

Approves credit arrangements with patients.

Reviews all accounts for referral to outside collection agencies prior to submission to the Business Office Manager.

Maintains and supervises all open patient accounts.

Performs any other duties requested by the Business Office Manager.

Qualifications

High school graduate with two years' college preferred.

One year hospital billing business office experience. Comparable experience with Blue Cross or other third party intermediary will be considered.

Participant in special workshops or training sessions in Medicare, Medicaid, and Blue Cross procedures to maintain a current, knowledgeable position relative to these procedures.

Knowledge of automated systems preferred.

Director of Admissions

Identification

Title: Director of Admissions

Department: Business Office

Supervisor: Business Office Manager

Position Description

Position Summary

Supervises Emergency Room Supervisor (if facility has that position), emergency room and outpatient registration areas, inpatient registration personnel, insurance verification staff (if separate positions), PBX operation, information desk, cashier, and transportation personnel (when applicable).

Duties and Responsibilities

Responsible for operation of the registration office and outpatient registration areas.

Monitors the creation, maintenance, and distribution of all required documents and statistical reports related to patient information.

Responsible for maintenance of patient and medical staff good will and the confidentiality of records.

Supervises reporting areas for department personnel to ensure appropriate staffing by function.

Establishes and maintains a pre-registration program, utilizing telephone and mail techniques. Communicates deposit requirements to patients and schedules registrations.

Supervises verification of insurance benefits, estimation of self-pay amounts due, and collection of registration deposits.

Responsible for an accurate bed control board and supporting procedures (if applicable) to maximize efficient registrations.

Responsible for maintenance of current and accurate registration logs.

Interviews patient or guarantor to obtain identifying and biographical information. Interprets hospital regulations to patients. Communicates rates, charges, services, discounts, and hospital policy regarding payment of bills.

Verifies compliance with hospital policies and procedures relative to registration practices.

Monitors cash collections and compliance with payment policies.

Monitors the patient's valuables procedures.

Conducts periodic staff meetings to inform staff of changes in registration office policies and procedures.

Reviews all admitting and registration folders daily.

Reviews all productivity reports daily.

Reviews pre-admission report and makes all necessary corrections or revisions weekly.

Makes rounds through all reporting areas daily.

Qualifications

High school graduate with one to two years' college preferred.

Minimum of two years' experience in a hospital registration office.

Knowledge of third party payors and insurance verification requirements required.

Billing Supervisor

Identification

Title: Insurance Billing Supervisor

Department: Business Office

Supervisor: Assistant Business Office Manager or Business Office Manager, as appropriate

Position Description

Position Summary

Has overall responsibility for submission of properly executed claims on a timely basis to guarantors, insurance carriers and intermediaries, performing rebilling and logging functions.

Duties and Responsibilities

Supervises and assists when necessary in submission of claims on a timely basis (average no more than six days after date of discharge or date of service).

Supervises and maintains follow-up procedure to secure approvals to bill Medicare and Medicaid accounts on a timely basis.

Trains new employees and holds periodic in-house training sessions. Requires thorough cross-training of employees to bill all types of coverage regardless of departmental organization.

Maintains diagnosis follow-up procedure and working relationship with Medical Records Director and physicians.

Maintains Daily Billing Productivity Report that includes detail type coverage and reason(s) for unbilled claims. Submits weekly summary to Business Office Manager.

Reviews in-house patient listing daily and directs interim billing in accordance with hospital procedures.

Reviews all problem bills to determine reason(s) for and resolution of problems, and delegates back to billers for billing.

Supervises logging procedures and ascertains that logs are kept current at all times.

Supervises handling of inquiries from carriers and patients regarding insurance claims and ascertains that they are answered correctly and timely.

Supervises timely preparation of input documents and submission to data processing.

Performs other duties as assigned by the Business Office Manager.

Qualifications

High school graduate with two years' college preferred.

One year hospital billing or business office experience. Comparable experience with Blue Cross or other third party intermediary will be considered.

Attendance at special workshops or training sessions in Medicare, Medicaid, and Blue Cross procedures to maintain current knowledge relative to these procedures.

Thorough knowledge of claims submission process for all major carriers and intermediaries.

Experience with on-line input terminal equipment and automated systems preferred.

Type a minimum of 40 w.p.m.

Admitting/Outpatient Registrar

Identification

Title: Admitting/Outpatient Registrar

Department: Admitting

Supervisor: Director of Admissions

Position Description

Position Summary

Responsible for registration of patients, including patient interviews, typing, room assignment and insurance verification; explanation of hospital policies regarding visitation, payment for charges, and services available. Handles routine patient inquiries and problems.

Duties and Responsibilities

Processes patient registrations in a timely and accurate fashion.

Promotes a positive hospital image of patients and physicians.

Receives and interviews incoming patients or relatives to obtain pertinent data.

Arranges for proper bed assignment according to patient type and diagnosis. Secures transportation services for patient.

Processes pre-registration documents.

Confirms insurance benefits, calculates and collects registration deposits.

Keys facesheet information and obtains patient's or responsible person's signature; creates arm bands, charge plates, and other documents as necessary.

Distributes registration records to business office, medical records, and ancillary departments.

Records each registration in log.

Collects patient valuables, depositing them for safekeeping and issues the patient a receipt.

Notifies nursing services and arranges for escort of patient to room (inpatient) and directs patient to appropriate ancillary department (outpatient).

Makes necessary changes on computer (insurance status, room changes), if applicable.

Ensures all patient files exist.

Ensures patient files are in order and forwarded to Director of Admissions the next day by 9:00 A.M.

Maintains pre-registration file.

Performs other duties as assigned by Supervisor.

Qualifications

High school diploma is required. One to two years' college preferred.

One year experience in a hospital, similar medical facility, or physician office preferred.

Experience with automated systems preferred.

Overall knowledge of business office procedures and hospital policies.

Knowledge of third party payors.

Type a minimum of 50 w.p.m.

Capable of operating 10-key calculator.

Excellent communication skills.

Emergency Room Registrar

Identification

Title: Emergency Room/Outpatient Registrar

Department: Business Office

Supervisor: Emergency Room Supervisor or Director of Admissions, as appropriate

Position Description

Position Summary

Registers emergency room patients for treatment, verifies insurance, calculates charges, collects payment for services, and directs patients to proper area for treatment.

Duties and Responsibilities

Responsible for prompt, courteous reception and processing of all patients presenting themselves for treatment.

Responsible for accurate and complete collection of registration data, charges, and cash payments.

Completes registration documents for emergency room patients on presentation of the patient in the emergency room.

Calculates all charges, reviews trial balances for unpaid, open, or written off accounts, and presents the patient with an itemized bill. Explains the hospital's policy regarding payment at time of service.

Receives payment in full for amount owed via cash, check, bank cards, or special financing.

Gathers insurance information, signatures, and forms needed to submit billings to third party payor for whom coverage is known.

Advises the admitting department of emergency inpatient registrations.

Records all patients seen on registration logs.

Deposits receipts to the main cashier daily and reconciles cash funds.

Ensures all patient files exist.

Ensures patient files are in order and forwarded to E.R. Supervisor or Director of Admissions, as applicable, by 9:00 A.M. the next day.

Performs other duties as assigned by E.R. Supervisor.

Qualifications

High school diploma required. One to two years of college preferred.

One year experience in a hospital, similar medical facility, or physician's office preferred.

Overall knowledge of business office procedures and hospital policies.

Knowledge of third party payors.

Experience with automated systems preferred.

Type a minimum of 50 w.p.m.

Capable of operating 10-key calculator.

Excellent communication skills.

Insurance Verifier

Identification

Title: Insurance Verifier

Department: Admitting

Supervisor: Director of Admissions

Position Description

Position Summary

Verifies third party payor and worker's compensation for all inpatients and outpatients.

Duties and Responsibilities

Verifies all third party payor and worker's compensation accounts.

Assists in registration process, as required.

Provides insurance information to physicians as requested.

Reviews patient folders for accuracy.

Documents information completely in the file.

Performs other duties as assigned by supervisor.

Qualifications

High school diploma required. One to two years of college preferred.

Knowledge of third party payors. One year admitting and/or insurance billing experience in a hospital, similar medical facility, or physician's office preferred.

Overall knowledge of business office procedures and hospital policies.

Capable of operating 10-key calculator.

Experience with automated systems preferred.

Type a minimum of 50 w.p.m.

Excellent communication skills.

Insurance Billing Clerk

Identification

Title: Billing Clerk

Department: Business Office

Supervisor: Billing Supervisor, Assistant Business Manager, or Business Office Manager, as appropriate

Position Description

Position Summary

Responsible for accurate and timely preparation and submission of claims to third party carriers and intermediaries, and answering inquiries on a timely basis according to hospital written procedures; for assigned section of alphabet.

Duties and Responsibilities

Responsible for maintenance and control of unbilled insurance file for a given section of patient accounts.

Reviews files daily and spot checks final bills for accuracy and readiness for billing.

Prepares and submits claims to carriers and intermediaries within 24 hours after all information is available for billing.

Prepares and submits a daily listing of all unbillable claims along with reason(s) to the Billing Supervisor or Business Office Manager by 10:00 A.M.

Prepares and submits daily input forms relative to billing function to data processing.

Prepares daily billing report.

Responsible for accurate accounting of all claims.

Performs other duties as assigned by Billing Supervisor or Business Office Manager.

Qualifications

High school diploma is required. One to two years of college preferred.

Knowledge of third party payors. Minimum six months' experience in hospital insurance billing or one year experience with major carrier in claims processing area.

One year experience in a hospital, similar medical facility, or physician's office preferred.

Overall knowledge of business office procedures and hospital policies.

Ability to type at least 50 w.p.m.

Capable of operating or learning to operate on-line input terminal.

Thorough knowledge of claims submission process for all major carriers and intermediaries.

Capable of operating 10-key calculator.

Excellent communication skills.

Collection Representative

Identification

Title: Collection Representative

Department: Business Office

Supervisor: Business Office Manager or Assistant Business Office Manager, as appropriate

Position Description

Position Summary

Responsible for implementing collection policies and procedures, interviewing and counseling patients, and other duties as assigned.

Duties and Responsibilities

Reviews delinquent account records and sends collection letters as needed according to written hospital procedures.

Answers debtor correspondence concerning delinquent accounts.

Monitors and continuously implements precollect program.

Telephones debtors and obtains payment or financing arrangements in accordance with written hospital procedures.

Maintains tickler file of accounts, following up by telephone or correspondence on outstanding balances.

Responsible for telephone and mail follow-up on amounts due from third party carriers on a timely basis in accordance with written hospital procedures.

Refers accounts to Business Office Manager on a weekly basis for write-off and agency or attorney referral.

Coordinates activities, answers inquiries, and provides documentation requested by collection agencies and attorneys.

Generates input documents and maintains bad debt files.

Assists in interviewing patients and obtaining financing, obtaining assistance in qualifying patients for Medicaid coverage, etc., and collecting all outstanding amounts.

Qualifications

High school diploma is required. One to two years of college preferred.

Six months-plus hospital business office experience; or at least one year experience in collection field. Proven sales ability considered a plus.

Overall knowledge of business office procedures and hospital policies.

General knowledge of third party payors, collection laws, F.T.C. rulings, and collection procedures.

Experience with automated system preferred.

Type a minimum of 50 w.p.m.

Capable of operating a 10-key calculator.

Excellent telephone communication skills.

Cashier

Identification

Title: Cashier

Department: Business Office

Supervisor: Business Office Manager

Position Description

Position Summary

Prepares hospital receipts for bank depositing and data entry; collects accounts and performs other business office control and review functions.

Duties and Responsibilities

Responsible for collection of daily mail from post office.

Responsible for the timely, intact, and accurate processing of hospital cash. Required to report violations of performance standards occurring in other departments turning in cash.

Responsible for verification that all control functions assigned are maintained daily.

Receives mail remittances and related information daily, records proper account numbers to each remittance, and prepares for data processing entry. Reviews third party vouchers for accurate account numbers and prepares for data processing entry.

Prepares and delivers daily bank deposits for all window, mail, outpatient, dietary, bad debt, and miscellaneous remittances.

Batches all cash for data entry and controls the daily bank deposits. Maintains a departmental cash batch log, along with a copy of the control sheet and balances to bank deposit and data transmittal acceptance notification daily.

Responsible for postage meter in the business office, replenishing it as necessary and controlling use.

Processes patient refunds and works credit balances.

Qualifications

High school graduate with a business/math emphasis preferred.

A minimum of one year business office experience.

Experience with automated systems preferred.

Type a minimum of 50 w.p.m.

Capable of operating a 10-key calculator.

Excellent communication skills.

File Clerk

Identification

Title: File Clerk

Department: Business Office

Supervisor: Assistant Business Office Manager or Business Office Manager, as appropriate

Position Description

Position Summary

Responsible for the accurate maintenance of various files in the business office. Controls receipt of registration documents and associated materials. Distributes materials within the department and locates materials as needed by area employees.

Duties and Responsibilities

Retains business office records in readily retrievable fashion.

Controls receipt and proper distribution of all materials required by department employees.

Distributes complete folders to the appropriate patient account billing clerk and files billed accounts in the proper file.

Distributes departmental mail and locates folders needed to respond to correspondence.

Receives and distributes telephone calls and patients to proper collection representative.

Pulls 1–31 cards, runs inquiries, and pulls corresponding accounts over $15; or pulls patient folders off computerized follow-up reports, as applicable, for collection representatives.

Copies and files EOB's for government programs in the patient folders.

Qualifications

High school diploma or equivalent required.

No previous experience is necessary; entry level position.

Alphabetizing skill.

Switchboard Operator

Identification

Title: Switchboard Operator

Department: Business Office

Supervisor: Director of Admissions or Business Office Manager, as appropriate

Position Description

Position Summary

Operates switchboard to relay incoming calls, outgoing calls, and pages. Screens visitors and releases patient condition information when authorized.

Duties and Responsibilities

Processes incoming and outgoing telephone calls efficiently, politely, and as quickly as possible.

Pages medical staff, surgical teams, disaster and emergency codes with dispatch and clarity in a calm manner.

Releases patient information as permitted by hospital policy.

Refers to hospital directory, determines station number of person being called, and connects caller as quickly as possible.

Places all long distance calls for patients and visitors.

Pages authorized personnel. Announces the close of visiting hours.

Greets and directs guests.

Maintains a trouble log for telephone equipment changes.

As backup for Admitting, performs discharges, mails datamailers, assists in pulling folders for the next day's collection follow-up, assists in outpatient billing and routine filing, as appropriate.

Assists the business office by breaking apart daily bills, making financial class and address changes, completing adjustment sheet for bad debt accounts, mailing self-pay bills, and so forth.

Performs other duties as assigned.

Qualifications

High school diploma required.

Previous experience as an operator or receptionist desirable.

Typing skills a plus.

Excellent communication skills.

Physical Requirements

Administrators may want to include physical requirements in certain job descriptions.

Class I—Light Physical Requirements

- Must be able to lift up to 25 pounds.
- Must be able to stand/walk for short periods of time.
- May be required to climb ladders/stools to heights of 3 feet or more.
- Must have full use of hands and arms, i.e., to operate typewriter, adding machine.
- Must be able to stoop and pick up objects from floor without restrictions.

Class II—Medium Physical Requirements

- Must be able to lift 60 pounds.
- Must be able to walk/stand without restrictions.
- Must be able to stoop and pick up objects from floor without restrictions.
- May be required to climb ladder/stool to height of 3 feet or more.
- Must have full use of both hands and arms with full range of movement.
- May not have hearing loss greater than 40 decibels.
- May not have vision loss greater than 20/40 (may be corrected with glasses or contact lenses).

Class III—Heavy Physical Requirements

- Must be able to lift 100 pounds or more.
- Must be able to walk/stand without restriction of any kind.
- Must be able to stoop and pick up objects from floor, including small items such as hypodermic needles, without restrictions.
- May be required to climb ladder/stool to height of 8 feet or more.
- Must have full use of both hands and arms with full range of movement.
- May not have hearing loss greater than 40 decibels.
- May not have vision loss greater than 20/40 (may be corrected with glasses or contact lenses).

B

Sample Miscellaneous Forms

The following form is required by Medicare and must be completed for every Medicare patient. The purpose of the form is to determine the primary carrier, and the form must be made available to Medicare upon request. Some fiscal intermediaries require the use of a different MSP form.

Medicare Secondary Payor—Inpatient/Outpatient Screening Form

PATIENT NAME: ______________________________

MEDICARE NO: ____________________ SERVICE DATES: ____________________

Ask all questions of each Medicare patient. If the patient responds "yes" to any question, ask the other applicable questions in that section. Please see the note at the bottom of the page. Have the patient or representative sign this form whenever possible.

Illness/Injury Caused by Accident

1. Is the illness or injury due to *any kind* of accident?

   [ ] No—Proceed with question #2 below.

   [ ] Yes—Medicare may be secondary. Check/complete the appropriate box (A–E).

A [ ] Motor Vehicle: Name of Patient's automobile insurer ____________________
Automobile Insurance is Primary: Bill them.

B [ ] Motor Vehicle: Name of Third Party's liability insurer ____________________
Liability may be Primary. Bill Medicare (unless patient's automobile insurer can pay first) and send copies of all pertinent documentation.

C [ ] Work Related: Name of Worker's Compensation insurer ____________________
Worker's Comp. insurance is primary. Bill them.

D [ ] Slip and Fall: Explain where fall occurred ____________________
____________________ If fall occurred at place other than patient's home, determine if liability claim or suit will be filed or if any kind of compensation can be made. Yes ____ No ____ (If yes, explain: Give information on third party insurer ____________________
____________________ Bill Medicare and send copies of all pertinent documentation.

E [ ] Other Accident, No Third Party Can Pay: Give description of accident and location ________
____________________ Bill Medicare and send copies of all pertinent documentation.

Coverage Through Other Government Entity

2. Does the Patient have coverage through the VA, Dept. of Labor's Black Lung Program, or some other federal or state agency program?

   [ ] No—Proceed with question #3 below.

   [ ] Yes—The entity the patient has coverage with must be billed primary to Medicare. Medicare may reject the claim unless the entity pays as primary or submits a denial of the services.

Employer Group Coverage for Those 65 and Over

3. Is the patient 65 or over and employed at the time of this service?

   [ ] No—Proceed with question #4 below.
   [ ] Yes—Give the patient's date of birth
   (MM/DD/YY) ________
   Give the name of the patient's company/employer ________________________

   A. Does the employer employ 20 or more employees?
      [ ] No [ ] Yes
   B. Does the patient have an Employer Group Health Plan (EGHP) by reason of his/her current employment?
      [ ] No [ ] Yes If yes, give the name of the EGHP
      ________________________ If the patient is aged 65 or over and has answered yes to A and B, the EGHP shown is primary to Medicare. Bill them first.

4. Does the patient have a spouse who is employed at the time of this service?

   [ ] No—Proceed with question #5 below.
   [ ] Yes—Give the *patient's* date of birth
   (MM/DD/YY) ________
   Give the name of spouse's company/employer ________________________

   A. Does the employer employ 20 or more employees?
      [ ] No [ ] Yes
   B. Does the spouse have an EGHP by reason of his/her current employment that covers the patient as a dependent? [ ] No [ ] Yes If yes, give the name of the EGHP ________________________
      If the patient is aged 65 or over and has answered yes to A and B, the EGHP shown is primary to Medicare. Bill the EGHP first.

Employer GRP Cov. for Those Entitled to M/Care Solely Due to ESRD

5. Is the patient under the age of 65, entitled to Medicare *solely* because of End Stage Renal Disease (ESRD), and in the first 12 months of Medicare entitlement?

   [ ] No—proceed with question 6 below.
   [ ] Yes—Give the patient's date of entitlement as shown on the Medicare Card (MM/YY) ________

   Does the patient have coverage through his/her, his/her spouse's, a parent's, or a guardian's EGHP?
   [ ] No [ ] Yes—Name of employer ________________________
   Name of EGHP ________________________

   If the patient answered yes to both questions, the EGHP is primary to Medicare. Bill them first. Medicare is secondary.

Employer GRP Coverage for Those Entitled to M/Care Solely Due to Disability

6. Is the patient under the age of 65, entitled to Medicare *solely* (does not have/has not had ESRD) because of disability?

   [ ] No—proceed to question #7.

   [ ] Yes—give the patient's date of birth (MM/DD/YY) ________________

   Does the patient have coverage through his/her, his/her spouse's, a parent's, or a guardian's EGHP?

   [ ] No [ ] Yes—Give name of each insured whose policy covers the patient

   a. ________________________ b. ________________________

   Give name of corresponding employer

   a. ________________________ b. ________________________

   Give name of corresponding EGHP

   a. ________________________ b. ________________________

   If the patient answered yes to both questions, the EGHP(s) is/are primary to Medicare. Bill the EGHP first.

7. Has the patient been an INPATIENT in a health care facility in the past 60 days?

   [ ] No—proceed with question #8 below.

   [ ] Yes—Complete "Prior Stay Information" below

   Facility Name ____

   Facility Type: Acute __ Skilled Nursing (SNF) __ Psych __

   Service Dates: Admit ____________________ Discharged ____________________

8. Does the patient belong to an HMO?

   [ ] No [ ] Yes—Obtain proper authorization form from HMO. (Medicare is not primary.) Is patient paying any insurance premiums? [ ] No [ ] Yes

   NOTE: It is important to ask all questions and document all answers regarding MSP. A provider may be held liable if an overpayment occurs and Medicare finds that the provider furnished erroneous information or failed to disclose facts relevant to payment. [Patient signature is on file]

Your Rights as a Medicare Patient

The following letter must be given to all Medicare patients as a directive from Health Care Financing Administration (HCFA) and can be on hospital letterhead.

An Important Message from Medicare

Your Rights While a Medicare Hospital Patient

- You have a right to receive all of the hospital care that is necessary for the proper diagnosis and treatment of your illness or injury. *Your discharge date should be determined solely by your medical needs,* not by "DRGs" or by Medicare payments.
- You have the right to be fully informed about decisions affecting your Medicare coverage or payment for your hospital stay.
- You have a right to appeal any *written* notices you receive from the hospital or Medicare stating that Medicare will no longer pay for your care.

Talk to Your Doctor

You and your doctor know more about your condition and your health care needs than anyone else. If you have questions about your medical treatment, your need for continued hospital care, or your discharge date, consult your doctor. These decisions should be made between you and your doctor. If you have questions or concerns about hospital services, you should talk to the hospital's patient representative or discharge planner. *Don't hesitate to ask questions*—you and your family should ask about your case, your stay in the hospital, and your planned discharge.

Peer Review Organizations

Peer Review Organizations (PROs) are groups of doctors who are paid by the federal government to review medical necessity, appropriateness, and quality of hospital treatment furnished to Medicare patients. Peer Review Organizations will respond to your request for review and appeal of written notices stating that Medicare will no longer pay for your stay.

If You Think You Are Being Asked to Leave the Hospital Too Soon

- Ask a hospital representative for a *written* notice of explanation *immediately,* if you have not already received one. The hospital's written notice is necessary if you decide to appeal to the PRO. The written notice must describe how you appeal.
- *If you decide to appeal, do so immediately—either call or write the PRO.* If you lose the appeal, you may be billed for all costs of stay beginning with the third day after you receive the written notice. The appeals process can take up to three *working* days from the time your appeal request is received. Thus, if you appeal and lose, you may have to pay for at least one day of hospital cost.
- REMEMBER: WITHOUT A WRITTEN NOTICE, YOU HAVE NO RIGHT TO APPEAL.

The Peer Review Organization for this area is: ____________________

ADDRESS: ____________________

____

____

TELEPHONE: ____________________

The following letter is completed and given to the patient when special financial arrangements are approved on a patient account. For example: The hospital will accept 80% coverage and waive the patient balance.

Dear ___________________________________:

(Hospital Name) is continuously striving to provide the most efficient and effective care possible. We hope your stay will be a pleasant one.

The following financial arrangements have been made to reduce your portion of liability on account # __________.

Arrangements: ____

____

____

Any deductible is to be paid on admission or prior to discharge.

The above financial arrangement pertains to *hospital charges* only and does not pertain to anesthesiology, radiology, pathology, or physician charges. *These arrangements do not apply to any insurance deductibles.*

Please note that any complication or unforeseen events in your care will void these arrangements. In such cases, all deposits paid will be applied to your account with the balance due on discharge. Your signature below signifies that you have understood and agree to these arrangements and terms.

Sincerely,

Director of Admissions

____ ____________________

Patient Signature (required) Date

Original: folder Copy: patient

____ ____________________

Admitting Representative Date

The following form should be completed when the hospital is requested to accept less than 100 percent payment for services rendered, and must be approved by administration. Once the arrangements are approved, the Financial Arrangements Letter should be completed and given to the patient.

Financial Arrangement Request

I/P __________ O/P __________

Patient Name: ______________________________ Phone: ______________________________

Physician Name: ______________________________ Phone: ______________________________

Diagnosis: ____

Procedure: ____

Request Date: ________ Admit Date: ________ Surgery Date: ______________________

Insurance Carrier: ____

Policy #/Group #: ____

Employer Name: ______________________________ Phone: ______________________________

Verified Coverage: ____

Requested:	________	Approved:	________ Medicare Only
	________		________ Medicare and Supplemental
	________		________ Insurance Only
	________		________ Insurance Only at 80% coverage*
	________		________ HMO/PPO Contract Benefits (If hospital is non-contracted)
	________		________ Misc: ______________

____

____

Approved by Administration   Date

*Patient is responsible for all deductibles.

The following form should be completed for any diagnosis related to mental health or to alcohol or drug abuse. This separate form is necessary to allow the hospital to release information to the insurance company or payor. The routine release of information form is not sufficient.

Release of Information

I, ______________________________, hereby authorize
Print: Last name, First, Middle Initial

(Hospital Name) to disclose medical records or other information

obtained for ______________________________
Print: Last name, First, MI

in the course of my/their diagnosis and treatment at said facility and as those records or information may pertain to mental health, alcohol, or drug abuse, to:

____

(Name of person or organization to which disclosure is made)

and the disclosure of records authorized herein is required for the following purpose: Discharge of the legal or contractual obligations of the third party payor or funding source,

and such disclosure shall be limited to the following specific type(s) of information: Admitting diagnosis, discharge diagnosis, history and physical, discharge summary progress notes

This consent is subject to revocation by the undersigned at any time except to the extent that action has been taken in reliance thereon, and not earlier revoked. It shall terminate on __________ without express revocation.
date

DATE: ____________________

____
Signature of Patient

WITNESS: ____________________

____
Date of Birth

____
Signature of parent, guardian, or authorized rep. of patient

____
E.R. Representative

____
Date

The following form is completed and signed by the patient whenever the "AIDS" test is administered to allow the hospital to release the results of the test to the payor. If the patient pays the charges in full, the form is not required.

Authorization for Disclosure of the Results of the HTLV-III Antibody Blood Test

This authorization for use or disclosure of the results of a blood test to detect antibodies to the Human Immunodeficiency Virus (HIV), the probable causative agent of Acquired Immune Deficiency Syndrome (AIDS), is being requested of you to comply with the terms of the Confidentiality of Medical Information Act, Civil Code Section 56 et seq. and Health and Safety Code Section 199.21(g).

I hereby authorize (Hospital Name) to furnish to:

____

(Name or title of person who is to receive results)
the results of the blood test for antibodies to the HIV.

The requester may use the information for any purpose, subject only to the following limitations: ____________

____

This authorization shall become effective immediately and shall remain in effect indefinitely, or until ________,

19 _____, whichever is shorter.

I understand that the requester may not further use or disclose the medical information unless another authorization is obtained from me or unless such use or disclosure is specifically required or permitted by law.

I further understand that I have a right to receive a copy of this authorization on my request.

Copy requested and received: _______ Yes _______ No Initial: _______

Date: ________________, 19 _________ ______________________________

Signature

____

Printed Name

The following form is completed and signed by the patient when the patient refuses to have blood administered. This form is sometimes maintained in the lab department because Admitting is not involved with the patient's status once admitted.

Refusal to Permit Blood Transfusion

I request that no blood derivatives be administered to ______________________________ during this hospitalization. I hereby release the hospital, its personnel, and the attending physician from any responsibility whatsoever for unfavorable reactions or any untoward results due to my refusal to permit the use of blood or its derivatives. The possible risks and consequences of such refusal on my part have been fully explained to me by my attending physician and I fully understand that such risks and consequences may occur as a result of my refusal.

______________________ Date

______________________ Patient/Parent/Conservator/Guardian

______________________ Time

If signed by other than patient, indicate relationship:

____

______________________ Witness

The following form is completed and signed by the patient when admitted as an "Overnight Guest."

Overnight Guest Program

Release Form

I have requested that (Hospital Name) permit me to stay the night before my procedure/surgery, which is to be performed on: date/time: ______________________________

I understand that the hospital *will not* offer any hospital, physician, or nursing services, except on an emergency basis, until two (2) hours prior to the time procedure/surgery is to be performed, as stated above. I therefore assume *all responsibility* for my stay at the hospital prior to this stated time and hereby release the hospital, its personnel, physicians, and other persons participating who are associated with the hospital from any liability for any harm or damages that may occur as a result of my stay at (Hospital Name) prior to my procedure/surgery.

I understand that this privilege is provided by (Hospital Name) for my convenience only and at no extra charge.

______________________	______________________	______________
Patient Signature	Today's Date	Time

Productivity Reports

The following reports are completed on a daily basis by each employee and are used as management tools to determine the quality of work performed and any problems encountered; they can be used to determine staffing levels.

Business Office Manager Checklist

The Business Office Manager checklist is a tool to assist the Business Office Manager in performing his or her primary duties. All of the activities on the checklist are completed either daily or weekly, depending on the activity.

Business Office Manager Checklist

Daily

_____ Review productivity reports

Business office
- _____ Billers
- _____ Medicare billing and follow-up
- _____ Medicaid billing and follow-up
- _____ Collectors
- _____ Correspondence

Admitting/ER registration
- _____ Admitting/Registration Clerk Activity
- _____ Financial counselling/In-house monitoring
- _____ Pre-admission
- _____ Insurance verification

_____ Review computer reports
- _____ Billing rejection
- _____ Unbilled report
- _____ ATB summary
- _____ Admission/Discharge/Transfer
- _____ Census
- _____ Batching reports
- _____ Error reports
- _____ Late charge reports

_____ Review admitting/registration folders

_____ Cash receipts. Obtain amount, record, and post in Business Office.

_____ Pending claims log

_____ Rounds made: _____ Admitting _____ PBX _____ Cashier _____ Business Office

Weekly

_____ Billing summary report distributed with unbillable logs

_____ Unbilled insurance report

_____ 240 report—Medicare

_____ Medical records request log

_____ Bad debt review/approval

_____ Random selection of accounts from each payor group reviewed
- _____ Is billing timely?
- _____ Is billing complete and accurate?
- _____ Is correspondence resolved?
- _____ Have contractuals been applied?
- _____ Is follow-up according to guidelines?
- _____ Has secondary insurance been billed?

_____ A/R Weekly Assessment completed and distributed

_______________________________ Clerk

_______________________________ Date

Admitting/Registration

Standard = 30 minutes per registration with verification; 15 minutes per registration without verification. (The entire registration process includes breaking the chart down, calculating deposit, etc.)

15 admits/registrations per day with verification
30 admits/registrations per day without verification

Number of admits ____________________

Number of pre-admits admitted ____________________

Number of outpatient registrations ____________________

Number of pre-admitted outpatients ____________________

Number of pre-admits ____________________

Number of telephone calls ____________________

Other:

____________________ ____________________

Clerk Date

E.R. Registration

Standard = 30 minutes per registration with verification; 15 minutes per registration without verification. (The entire registration process includes breaking the chart down, calculating deposit, etc.)

15 registrations per day with verification
30 registrations per day without verification

Number of registrations ____________________

Number of telephone calls received ____________________

Number of admits ____________________

Other:

Daily Billing Report

The daily billing report is a tool to measure employee productivity and analyze work flows. The Business Office Manager can determine if billers are meeting production goals (a biller should be able to bill an average of 50–80 clean claims per day). A biller is supposed to bill clean claims only; any claims that cannot be billed are to be notated on the pending claims log and referred to the Business Office Manager for review. A biller should be billing only—not answering telephones, pulling files, breaking apart bills, and so forth. The billing report documents all activities the billers are performing; therefore, it is designed to detect any activities or duties the billers perform that prevent maximization of production.

The billing report, along with the pending claims log, is to be turned into the Business Office Manager at the end of each day.

Beginning balance—Unbilled accounts from the previous day

New claims received—Accounts that dropped from the system that day

Total claims—Total claims to be billed

# of claims billed—Total number of claims billed

Ending balance—Number of claims to be billed (includes accounts on the pending claims log)

Rebills—Number of accounts rebilled

Secondary insurance—Number of secondary insurances billed

Comments—Used to document other activities performed and the time involved and any additional information

Daily Billing Report

Today's Date ____________________

Standard = 50 claims per day (one claim every 9 minutes) to begin; work up to 80 claims per day (approximately 1 claim every 5.5 minutes)

	Number of Accounts	*$ Amount of Accounts*
Beginning balance	______	______
New claims received	______	______
Total claims to be billed	______	______
Number of claims billed	______	______
Ending balance to be billed	______	______
Rebills	______	______
Secondary Insurance (X-overs)	______	______

Comments: ____

____

____

____

____

____

____

____

____

____

Employee Signature

____

Daily Billing Report (Example)

Today's Date ____________

Standard = 50 claims per day (one claim every 9 minutes) to begin; work up to 80 claims per day (approximately 1 claim every 5.5 minutes)

	Number of Accounts	*$ Amount of Accounts*
Beginning balance	150	$250,000
New claims received	75	100,000
Total claims to be billed	225	350,000
Number of claims billed	21	50,000
Ending balance to be billed	204	$300,000
Rebills		
Secondary Insurance (X-overs)		

Comments:

1. Had to correct 5 claims.
2. Billed three claims from scratch.
3. Broke apart bills from 8:00 A.M. to 10:00 A.M.
4. Answered 8 phone calls.
5. Talked to three patients regarding their bills.
6. Billed 10 self-pay and did my mail on postage machine (½ hour).
7. Did special project for business office manager—1 hour.

____

Employee Signature

Daily Billing Report Analysis (Example)

50 Goal

1. 21 Claims—189 minutes = 3 hours 9 minutes
2. Why did we have to correct 5 claims?
   A. Did Admitting miss code?
   B. Does the master plan need correcting?
3. Why did we bill three claims from scratch?
   A. See Item 2.
4. Why did it take 2 hours to break apart bills?
   A. Is profile same as pending bills?
   B. Can it be done by someone else?
5. Phone calls
   A. What kind of phone calls?
   B. Billers should not answer phones.
6. What was the problem with their bills?
   A. Were charges right?
   B. Is the description confusing?
   C. Were they coded right?
   D. Had we sent them an itemized statement?
   E. Should someone else be helping instead of the biller?
7. Late shifts or someone else should be able to bill self-pay and mail.
8. Need to be careful with special projects—Billing is behind.

Pending Claims Log

The pending claims log is a mechanism to document all accounts that have dropped from the computer system but, for some reason, are unable to be billed. The pending claims log, when used in conjunction with system-generated reports and reports of unbilled secondaries, supplemental, and rebillings, will give hospital management a total number and amount of unbilled claims.

The pending claims log also keeps billers' production high. Because billers should be working only on clean claims, the report creates a controlled atmosphere.

Billers document any account that they cannot bill onto the pending claims log. The logs should be cumulative, listing the current day's unbillable claims plus any previous claims that have not been billed. Pending claims logs, accompanied by the folders and bills, are turned into the Business Office Manager on a daily basis. The Business Office Manager should review the logs to analyze problems, such as incomplete registrations, medical records problems, etc., and determine a method for resolution of the problems.

Patient Name—Name of the patient

Account #—Number of account

Balance—Balance of account

Discharge date—Date of discharge

Diagnosis—Account is missing discharge diagnosis

Coding—Account is missing medical records codes

Phys—Physician's notes are missing

U.R.—Need U.R. information

Attest—Missing physician's attestation statement

Other—Account cannot be billed for other reasons

Comments—Explanation for other reasons and/or additional information

(List items that reflect problem areas the facility needs to track.)

The billers are to complete the pending claims log, total the amounts of unbillable accounts, and turn in to the Business Office Manager at the end of each day. The Business Office Manager can delegate problems back to the billers to resolve. The key issue is to control the problems and provide a mechanism for the Business Officer Manager to be made aware of problems on a consistent basis.

Date: ____________________

Name: ____________________

Pending Claims Log

Patient Name	Account #	Balance	Discharge Date	Diax	Coding	Phys	U.R.	Attest	Other	Comments

Date: ____________

Name: ____________

Pending Claims Log

Patient Name	Account #	Balance	Discharge Date	Diax	Coding	Phys	U.R.	Attest	Other	Comments
		2,500.00	10/01/84	X						
		3,000.00	09/30/84	X						
		2,000.00	10/15/84					X		
		1,000.00	10/20/84					X		
		1,000.00	10/05/84	X						
		4,000.00	10/03/84	X						
		5,000.00	10/01/84					X		
		2,000.00	10/05/84					X		
		10,000.00	09/25/84	X						
		8,000.00	09/28/84	X						
		6,000.00	10/07/84					X		
		4,000.00	10/20/84					X		
		3,000.00	10/15/84					X		
		5,000.00	10/04/84	X						
		7,000.00	09/30/84					X		
		2,000.00	10/07/84	X						
		2,000.00	10/15/84	X						
		4,000.00	10/10/84	X						
		5,000.00	10/09/84						X	Sterilization
		8,000.00	10/02/84						X	Sterilization
		1,000.00	10/16/84	X						
		4,000.00	10/06/84					X		
		6,000.00	08/15/84						X	Medical Necessity
		5,000.00	09/02/84						X	No Assignment
Totals		109,500.00		42,500				32,000	24,000	

Pending Claim Log Analysis

1. Figures can be used for unbilled on monthly operating report.
2. $109,500 unbilled representing several A/R days.
3. Account age is several weeks.
4. Three major problem areas exist.
   - A. Diax.—Medical records, doctors, or procedure
   - B. Attestations—physicians
   - C. Attachments:
     - 1) Physician inservice
     - 2) Procedures in admitting office

Insurance Verification Daily Report

The insurance verification daily report is designed to measure employee productivity, analyze work flows, monitor verification results, and identify problems that prevent timely and accurate verifications. The Director of Admissions and/or Business Office Manager can determine if all verifications are being performed on a timely basis to improve cash flow and minimize bad debts.

Personnel responsibility for performing the verification function is to complete a verification report daily, or it can be included as part of the Registrar's report if they perform the verification.

Insurance Verification Representative Daily Report

Minimum Beginning Standard = 40 verifications per day

Balance forward from yesterday I/P ____________ O/P ____________

Pre-admit verifications (received) I/P ____________ O/P ____________

Pre-admit verifications (completed) I/P ____________ O/P ____________

Other verifications received I/P ____________ O/P ____________

Other verifications completed I/P ____________ O/P ____________

Total verifications completed I/P ____________ O/P ____________

Ending balance I/P ____________ O/P ____________

Relief (time): ____________________ for whom: ____

Phone calls—Incoming: ____

Outgoing: ____

Special financing applications completed: ____

Have all pre-admits for tomorrow been financially cleared?
Yes No (circle one) If not, please state explanation under "Comments."

Comments: ____

____

____

____

____

____

Please complete, sign, and return to Director of Admissions on a daily basis. Use the comments section to describe any unusual occurrences and any possible problems that need addressing—include dates, times, and the names and departments of those involved.

Daily Collection Log

The daily collection log is designed to measure employee productivity, analyze work flow, and spot trends. The Business Office Manager can determine if collectors are reaching their production goals (a collector should have an average of 40 contacts per day) and are concentrating on high dollar accounts instead of expending efforts on low dollar accounts or uncollectible accounts.

It is also a control mechanism to ensure that follow-up is according to hospital guidelines and, when reviewed by the Business Office Manager with the employee, serves as a training tool.

Collection representatives use the collection logs daily to notate all follow-up contacts and any other activities they get involved with. They enter detail documentation on the file or in the computer system. Comments on the report should be very brief and made only when something doesn't apply to the pre-printed headings. The total dollar amounts of the accounts contacted are calculated, and the log turned in to the Business Office Manager at the end of each day. Patient folders and/or collection notes accompany the report. In addition to analyzing the collection logs, the Business Office Manager also reviews collection notes to ensure that quality contacts are being made.

Patient name—Name of the patient contacted

Account #—Patient's account number(s)

Balance—Balance of outstanding account(s)

P/P—Promise to pay—amount and date

N/A—No answer to telephone call

LMCO—Left message for patient to call office

SL—Sent letter to patient

Call In—Patient called into office

Other—Any other type of contact

Comments—Used to document explanation of "Other" and/or any additional information

Date: ______________________

Name: ______________________

Daily Collection Log

Patient Name	Account #	Balance	P/P	N/A	LMCO	SL	Call In	Other	Comments

Date: ____________

Name: ____________

Daily Collection Log

Patient Name	Account #	Balance	P/P	N/A	LMCO	SL	Call In	Other	Comments
		75.00			X				
		52.00		X		X			
		99.00			X				
		20.00		X		X			
		15.00					X		
		35.00					X		
		82.00		X		X			
		70.00			X		X		
		65.00		X		X			
		90.00					X		
		42.00					X		
		25.00					X		
		110.00	X						
		125.00	X						
		95.00		X		X			
		80.00			X				
		100.00	X						
	Spent 1 hour working on correspondence								
	Spent 1 hour 15 minutes taking care of problem accounts								
	Spent 30 minutes transferring charges from ER account to I/P account								

Daily Collection Log Analysis

40 Goal

1. 17 Calls = 204 minutes = 3 hours and 24 minutes.
2. All balances are small balances.
3. Large percentage of letters sent.
   - A. May need to have late shift.
   - B. Collectors may not be calling place of employment.
4. Left message contact office (See Item 3).
5. High percentage of call-ins.
   - A. What is causing the calls?
   - B. Is insurance behind?
   - C. Are data mailers profiled properly?
6. What kind of correspondence (See Item 5)?
   - A. Maybe some other person should be designated to handle.
7. Problem accounts.
   - A. How many?
   - B. What kind of problems?
   - C. What is causing the problem?
8. Charge transfer.
   - A. Why did this happen?
   - B. Is Nursing at fault or Admitting?
   - C. Is no one reviewing files?
9. Are collection files being reviewed daily to determine proper collection techniques that are being used?
10. 6 Hours 9 minutes accounted for.

Index

About the Author

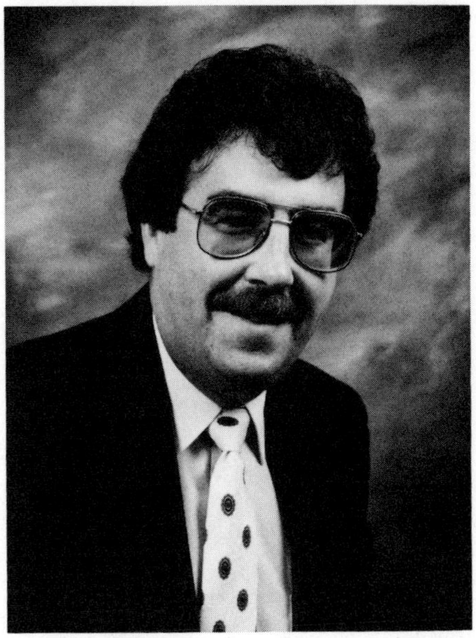

Dudley Medlock is owner and president of D-MED Corporation based in Dallas, Texas. D-MED Corporation is a business office and accounts receivable management and consulting firm with a national client base.

Mr. Medlock has more than eighteen years of management experience, with the past fourteen years in healthcare. His experience covers a broad spectrum of business office management issues. He has been a business office manager and director of business office services for a large proprietary chain. His experience has exposed him to for-profit as well as to not-for-profit facilities, small and large facilities, rural and urban facilities, and specialty facilities. He has served as a chapter president for a local Lions club and as district governor responsible for forty Lions clubs. He was also president of the Hawthorne chapter of AGPAM in Missouri for three years.

Mr. Medlock's travels and experience have given him an acute awareness of the difficulties facing today's director of patient accounting. Thus, he receives frequent requests for speaking engagements to address management issues in patient accounting.

Mr. Medlock is a member of HFMA and AGPAM, and he is a CPAM through the American Guild of Patient Account Management.

About the Author